Dad –

This book contains some good hints for emergency care. I also like its list of articles to have in a first aid kit. I hope you like it too.

Fondly,
Bonnie and
Family

W9-CKL-790

THE

FAMILY
FIRST AID
AND
MEDICAL
GUIDE

EMERGENCIES	IN THE HOME
SYMPTOMS	ON THE ROAD
TREATMENTS	ON VACATION

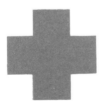

Dr James Bevan
MA, MB, BChir, MRCGP, DObst RCOG

Senior Medical Consultant to
The Automobile Association

SIMON AND SCHUSTER

Advisory Panel

R. W. Beard, MD, FRCOG,
Professor of Obstetrics and Gynaecology,
St Mary's Hospital, London

A. W. Boylston, MD, MRCPath,
Wellcome Senior Fellow in Clinical Science,
St Mary's Hospital Medical School, London

Anthony Catterall, MChir, FRCS,
Consultant Orthopaedic Surgeon,
Royal National Orthopaedic Hospital
and New Charing Cross Hospital, London

Dr R. M. Moffitt, MA, MB, MRCP, FRCGP, DO,
General Practitioner and Senior
Medical Officer, University of Lancaster

Dr J. F. Robinson, MB, ChB, MRCGP,
General Practitioner

Revised and expanded from the book originally published
in 1979 as *The Pocket Medical Encyclopedia and First
Aid Guide*
Edited and designed by
Mitchell Beazley International Limited
87–89 Shaftesbury Avenue, London W1V 7AD
This edition © Mitchell Beazley Publishers 1984
Text © Fennlevel Limited 1984
All rights reserved including the right of reproduction
in whole or in part in any form
Published by Simon and Schuster
A division of Simon & Schuster, Inc.
Simon & Schuster Building, Rockefeller Center
1230 Avenue of the Americas
New York, New York 10020
ISBN 0–671–50891–1
Filmsetting by Vantage Photosetting Co Ltd
Eastleigh, England
Origination by Nickeloid Litho Ltd, London
Printed and bound in Italy by New Inter Litho, Milan

Editor David Townsend Jones
Art Editor Jill Raphaeline

Executive Editor Susan Egerton-Jones
Editorial Assistant Rosemary Bevan
Artist Frank Kennard
Production Jean Rigby

Foreword

It is recognized by all that at one time or another we will be faced with a medical emergency – something that can happen at any time whether we are out on the road, away on vacation or at home. There are, too, those far more frequent occasions – a travel-sick child, a grazed knee, a wasp sting and so on – when positive, reliable response is all that is needed. I believe the reader will find confidence in using this book and in taking sensible, practical steps to cope with an emergency if and when it arises.

This book has been designed in three readily accessible sections. The opening FIRST AID section provides detailed advice on equipping a home medicine cabinet and a portable first aid kit for the car, followed by concise information on what to do at the scene of an accident and an illustrated step-by-step guide to life-saving techniques, complemented by an alphabetical directory of first aid treatments. The wide-ranging second section, HEALTH AND SAFETY, covers subjects such as vacation and travel preparations, helpful advice for safe motoring, accident prevention, emergency survival techniques and home care for the sick. MEDICAL ENCYCLOPEDIA, the final section, provides a complete medical reference: full-colour illustrations of how the human body works, charts of symptoms and how to assess them, information on medical words and medicinal drugs, plus a comprehensive, alphabetically organized directory of diseases, symptoms and treatments.

To the user it may appear that this book has been the work of one person – myself. Yet without the advice and professional assistance of others the book would not have been possible. The original *The Pocket Medical Encyclopedia and First Aid Guide* on which this handbook is based was edited by Hal Robinson and largely illustrated by Coral Mula. Their contributions have stood and continue to stand the test of time and use. To them I remain indebted. On this book I would particularly like to thank the editorial team at Mitchell Beazley, who are mentioned elsewhere, and also the artist, Frank Kennard; the Advisory Panel who checked the manuscript; Bill Halden and his staff at The Automobile Association, England, whose generous research made my life easier; and finally my wife, Rosemary, who helped me throughout with the manuscript.

James Bevan

CONTENTS

How to use this book   5

FIRST AID

Introduction   6
Home medicine cabinet   6
First aid kit   8
Action at a road crash   10
First aid at an accident   11
Life-saving   12
Alphabetical directory of problems and
    treatments   19

HEALTH AND SAFETY

Introduction   45
Fitness to travel   46
Keeping healthy on vacation   47
Car safety and kit   49
Accident procedures   51
Fitness to drive   52
Safety on two wheels   53
Camping   55
Hiking   58
Winter sports   59
Water sports   60
Survival techniques   61
Domestic accident prevention   66
Good health and fitness   68
Care of the sick at home   71

MEDICAL ENCYCLOPEDIA

Introduction   76
Medical words   76
How the body works – Anatomy and
    physiology   81
Symptoms: Charts of what to do   91
A–Z of diseases, symptoms and treatments   101
Medicinal drugs   168

INDEX   173

Country-by-country medical and
    motoring requirements   184
Family medical records   186
Emergency charts   191

How to use this book

The book is designed for quick and easy reference throughout. FIRST AID (p.6), HEALTH AND SAFETY (p.45) and MEDICAL ENCYCLOPEDIA (p.76) each opens with a short introduction summarizing the contents of the relevant section. Main cross-references to other parts of the book are always printed in a distinctive 'small capitals' typeface (e.g. 'see CARE OF THE SICK AT HOME'), while other methods of cross-referencing are clearly explained as they arise.

The pages of the FIRST AID section are colour-edged for rapid access (the emergency LIFE-SAVING pages in red, the ALPHABETICAL DIRECTORY of first aid treatments in pink) and every cross-reference to these throughout the book is printed in a distinctive red, with a page number (e.g. 'see FIRST AID: Sprain, p.42'). There is also a comprehensive INDEX.

For a quick step-by-step symptoms guide to what to do when a common problem (such as headache or sore throat) occurs, turn to the CHARTS OF WHAT TO DO on pp.91–100. A further useful feature is the inclusion of Checklists throughout the book, to remind you what to buy or pack, or carry with you on a journey.

Following the INDEX, at the back of the book, there are pages for information that only you can fill in: your FAMILY MEDICAL RECORDS and EMERGENCY CHARTS. Be sure to complete these so that this book can really work for you and your family.

FIRST AID

Introduction

This section tells you how to be equipped and prepared for emergencies and what to do if one occurs.

If no doctor is present at an emergency it is essential to do the right things as quickly as possible. This may save the victim's life. The FIRST AID AT AN ACCIDENT chart on p.11 shows what to do in any circumstances; in the event of a road accident it should be used in conjunction with the ACTION AT A ROAD CRASH chart on the opposite page (p.10). Remember that your life is important too – always try to get any help available and never take unnecessary risks.

First Aid techniques – the major subject of this section – are described in two parts. LIFE-SAVING (pp.12–18) shows with clear illustrations and simple explanations how to check for and restore the victim's breathing and heartbeat. The ALPHABETICAL DIRECTORY (pp.19–44) describes emergencies both major and minor that you may encounter and gives details of the necessary first aid treatment for each one.

There is also advice on organizing a HOME MEDICINE CABINET (pp.6–7) and on how to equip a FIRST AID KIT for your car (pp.8–9).

See also:
    SURVIVAL TECHNIQUES   pp.61–65
    ACCIDENT PROCEDURES pp.51–52

Home medicine cabinet

Keep a stock of medicines and basic accessories in a safe place, ideally in a cabinet specially designed with a childproof lock and well out of the reach of children. Do not use it to store anything except first aid equipment and medical drugs.

The cabinet should contain all medicines prescribed by a doctor as well as those purchased from a pharmacist. Pills should never be left by the bedside where children may find them. Unused drugs and medicines or those whose expiration date (usually written on the label) has passed should be returned to the pharmacist for disposal.

The following is a suggested checklist for your home medicine cabinet. When an article is used up it should be replaced immediately. All items recommended can be obtained from a pharmacist without a doctor's prescription.

If possible a first aid book should be kept in the cabinet. If there is not room, a safe place is on top where it can be reached when the cabinet is opened. Adult members of the family should be familiar with the book so that first aid, when it is needed, can be carried out both quickly and safely.

Checklist – First aid cabinet

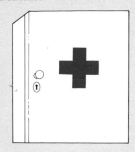

Emergency information, including the telephone number of your local doctor, hospital and pharmacist

Large, blunt-ended scissors

Square-ended tweezers for removing splinters

Clinical thermometer, kept in a case

Package of safety pins

Sterile absorbent cotton

Two 5cm (2ins) elastic (crepe) bandages

Two 7.5cm (3ins) elastic (crepe) bandages

Five sterile gauze dressings in individual packages

Four 5 × 5cm (2 × 2ins) non-adherent sterile dressings with perforated plastic coverings (for use on burns and scrapes)

One 10cm × 3m (4ins × 10ft) elastic adhesive bandage

Box of 7.5cm (3ins) adhesive dressing strips with central medicated gauze

Package or box of individual adhesive Band-Aids

One sterile eye pad

Two 2.5cm (1in) rolls of non-allergic surgical tape

Two triangular bandages (for use as slings)

Useful drugs in the home

Colds:	chlorpheniramine tablets; ephedrine nose drops (10ml bottle)
Constipation:	bisacodyl tablets; glycerine suppositories (package of 10)
Coughs:	proprietary cough mixture
Fever:	soluble aspirin tablets (300mg)
Diarrhea:	kaolin mixture (200ml); Loperamide capsules (2mg: package of 20)
Headaches/ pain:	codeine and acetaminophen tablets (bottle of 25)
Indigestion:	magnesium trisilicate mixture (200ml bottle); antacids
Rash/sunburn:	calamine lotion (200ml bottle)
Scrapes:	cetrimide cream
Sore throat:	benzalkonium lozenges (package of 25)
Wound cleaning:	hexachlorophene liquid (200ml bottle); topical antibiotic ointment

For babies and children

Rectal thermometer

One 200ml bottle of phenergan (for colds, travel sickness and night sedation)

One 100ml bottle of kaolin mixture for children (for diarrhea)

One 100ml bottle of acetaminophen mixture (for fever and pain)

One bottle of ephedrine nose drops for infants (for colds)

First aid kit

Checklist
1. Various sizes sterile dressings
2. One roll of adhesive tape
3. Eye pad with bandage
4. Sterile 10 × 10cm (4 × 4ins) gauze pads
5. Tube of antibiotic ointment
6. Box of assorted Band-Aids
7. Rolls of elastic (crepe) bandage
8. One roll of stretchable roller gauze
9. Two sterile triangular bandages, for slings
10. Several alcohol swabs
11. Several large safety pins
12. Blunt-ended scissors

The kit contains standard replaceable items available from any pharmacist. It should be kept in a safe place in the car, away from children and not on the rear window shelf where it may be thrown forward, hitting the passengers or driver if the car stops suddenly.

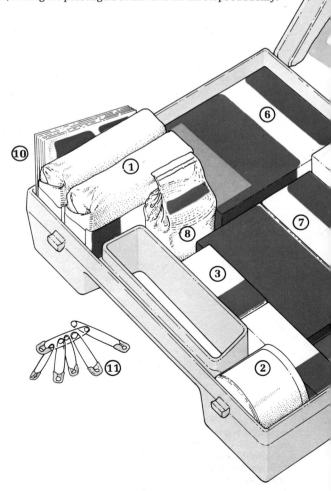

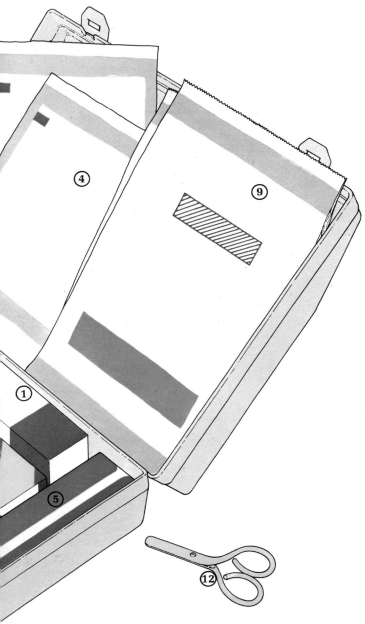

The contents of the first aid kit can be supplemented by several useful drugs such as those recommended in KEEPING HEALTHY ON VACATION: Checklist – Drugs for travelling abroad, p.48.

In addition to a first aid kit a fire extinguisher should be fitted to all cars that do not have one as standard. For further details about CAR SAFETY AND KIT, see pp.49–50.

Action at a road crash

1. Turn off car engine.

2. Switch on hazard warning lights.

3. No smoking! Extinguish all cigarettes, etc.

4. Assess need for **First aid at an accident** (see opposite). Treat most seriously injured first and always release motorcyclists' helmet straps, but **DO NOT** remove helmet.

5. If help available, send someone to:
Erect red warning flare about 10 metres (30 feet) behind accident to alert following traffic;
Alert oncoming traffic (preferably with second red warning flare if available); and:

6. Alert rescue and ambulance services.

See on pp.51–52 ACCIDENT PROCEDURES: Checklists – At a road accident; For injury at a road accident; For insurance claim.

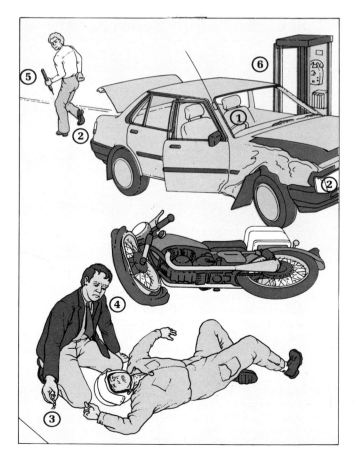

First aid at an accident

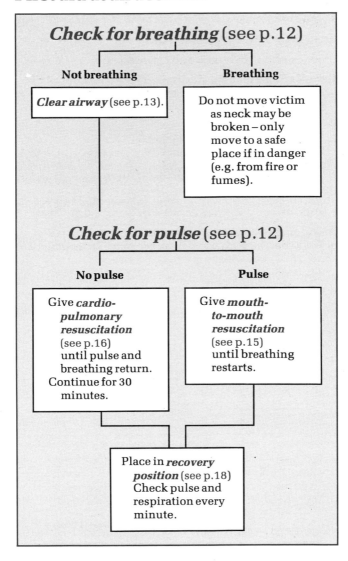

Check for breathing (see p.12)

Not breathing

Clear airway (see p.13).

Breathing

Do not move victim as neck may be broken – only move to a safe place if in danger (e.g. from fire or fumes).

Check for pulse (see p.12)

No pulse

Give *cardio-pulmonary resuscitation* (see p.16) until pulse and breathing return. Continue for 30 minutes.

Pulse

Give *mouth-to-mouth resuscitation* (see p.15) until breathing restarts.

Place in *recovery position* (see p.18) Check pulse and respiration every minute.

In all cases the casualty must lie on the floor

If **bleeding** – press on source of bleeding ... pp.21–22
If **bones fractured** – do not move the casualty ... p.30
If **burned** by fire – immerse in cold water ... p.23
If **burned** by liquids – remove soaked clothes ... p.23
If **choking** – force air out of the lungs ... pp.17–18
If **conscious** – keep the casualty talking ... pp.43–44
If having **convulsions** – do not restrict movement ... pp.25–26
If **poisoned** or **stung** – keep the casualty calm ... pp.40; 42–43
If **unconscious** – check pulse and breathing ... p.12

OBTAIN HELP AS SOON AS POSSIBLE

Life-saving
Checking for breathing and pulse

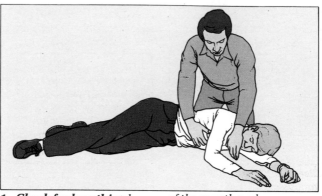

1. Check for breathing by placing your hand on the patient's chest and in front of the mouth and nose. Always call for medical assistance.

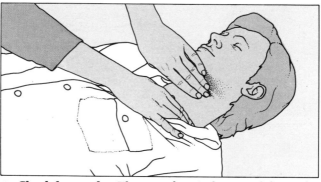

2. Check for a pulse. The strongest pulse is in the neck. It can be felt between the windpipe and the angle of the jaw. The pulse in the wrist is hard to detect.

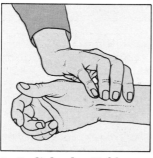

3. Radial pulse. Hold your fingers on the inside of the wrist in line with the thumb.

The carotid pulse in the neck gives the clearest indication that the heart is beating. It is often impossible to feel any pulse at all in the wrist of an injured person. The colour and feel of the patient's skin are other signs of cardiac arrest. The skin is likely to be gray and cold and the lips pale. If the heart is not beating, the patient needs heart massage (pp.13–14) at once.

Clearing the airway

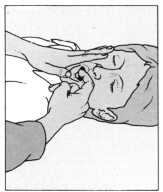

Clear the airway *and remove anything blocking the free flow of air.*

The patient must be turned face-up. Remove obstructions from the mouth by tilting the head to one side and holding the mouth open with your thumb. Use your other hand to remove anything, such as false teeth or a toy, that blocks the patient's throat. If the mouth is damaged, make sure that the nose is clear so that mouth-to-nose resuscitation (p.15) can be used. If this is not possible, see the Holger Nielsen or Silvester methods, pp.16–17.

Preparing for artificial respiration

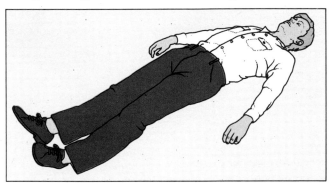

1. Lay the patient face-up *on a hard surface such as the floor for both heart massage and mouth-to-mouth artificial respiration. Loosen clothing around the neck.*

Heart massage

If the patient's heart has stopped, three quick, firm presses on the chest over the breastbone may start it beating again. If not, a steady, regular rhythm of one press a second is required.

This must be continued until the heart starts again or until medical help arrives.

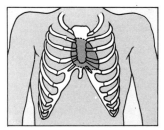

1. The heart *lies under the breastbone and towards the left of the patient's chest.*

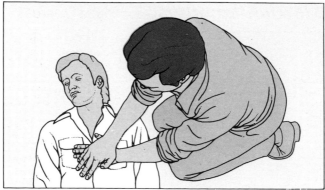

2. Heart massage. *Kneel at the patient's left shoulder. Place one hand on the other so that your fingers touch the bottom of the breast-bone. Press firmly with the whole of your hand evenly over the area of the heart.*

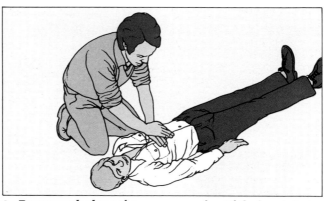

3. Press regularly *on the heart with one press a second until the heart starts to beat rhythmically again.*

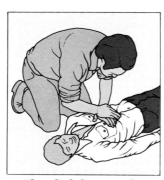

4. Flex slightly as you lean forward. *The chest compresses about 5cm (2 inches). Press gently on children.*

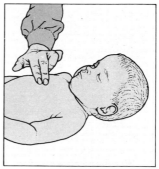

5. For a baby's heart, *it is sufficient to press with two fingers only, at approximately one hundred beats a minute.*

Mouth-to-mouth/nose resuscitation

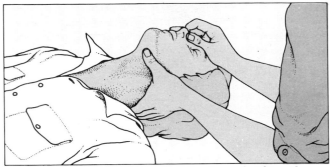

1. Prepare for mouth-to-mouth (or mouth-to-nose) resuscitation by lifting the patient's neck, tilting the head and pinching the nose.

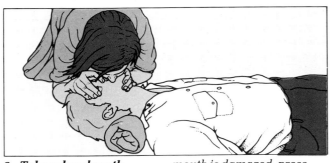

2. Take a deep breath. Cover the patient's mouth with your mouth. Blow steadily into the lungs. If the mouth is damaged, press firmly on the jaw to close it, and blow through the nostrils.

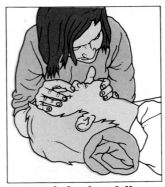 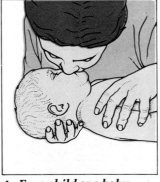

3. Watch the chest fall as you take another breath. If this fails, check that the airway is clear (see p. 13). Repeat the breath every five seconds.

4. For a child or a baby, cover both mouth and nose with your mouth and blow very gently, just enough to see the chest move. Repeat every three to four seconds.

Cardio-pulmonary resuscitation

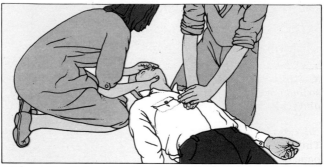

If the patient's heart has stopped, breathing will also cease. Combine heart massage with mouth-to-mouth or mouth-to-nose resuscitation.

This is easier if two people are present. One person kneels at the patient's left shoulder to give heart massage (pp.13–14) at the rate of one press a second. The other person kneels at the patient's right side to give mouth-to-mouth resuscitation (p.15) every five seconds. If you are alone give five heart massages and then one mouth-to-mouth respiration. This should continue for at least half an hour after the heart has stopped or until the patient is breathing normally.

Artificial respiration, alternative methods

Mouth-to-mouth resuscitation (p.15) is the most effective method for restarting breathing. If the mouth and nose are damaged it is not practicable, however, and in such cases the Holger Nielsen or Silvester methods should be used.

Holger Nielsen method
The patient must be lying face-down. Kneel at the head and lean over so that your hands rest on the patient's shoulder blades.

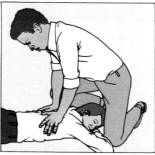 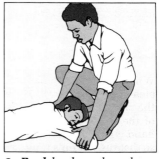

1. Press on the shoulder blades to expel the air from the patient's lungs.

2. Rock backwards and hold the patient's elbows. Raise them from the ground.

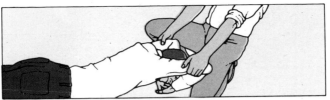

3. Lift the patient's elbows so that the chest expands and sucks in air.

4. Lower the elbows, and repeat the cycle once every five seconds.

Silvester method

This is used when the patient is lying face-up. Heart massage (pp.13–14) can be given at the same time. To do this, press firmly on the heart once a second when the patient's arms are raised. One person can combine heart massage with artificial respiration if ten presses on the heart are given between each cycle of the Silvester method, but the combination is easier with two people.

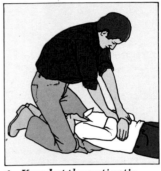

1. Kneel at the patient's head, hold the wrists and press on the rib cage.

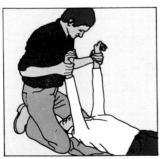

2. Raise the arms upwards and bring them outwards and down by your side.

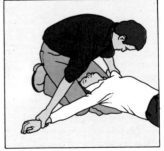

3. This expands the lungs and sucks air in. Repeat the cycle every five seconds.

Choking

When a person chokes, the blocked air passage must be cleared immediately. When an adult starts to choke, grasp the victim from behind. Clench one hand below the bottom of the rib cage (over the midriff) and hold this clenched hand with the other hand. Pull the hands sharply upwards so that the victim's lungs are compressed and the air expelled forcibly from them. This process, the Heimlich maneuver, is intended to dislodge the blockage. Artificial respiration (pp.13–17) may then be needed.

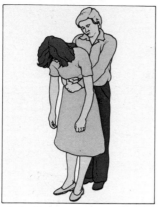

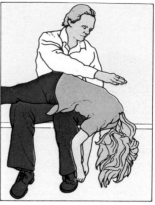

Heimlich maneuver. *Hold one hand in the other and pull sharply upwards to compress the lungs.*

For a child, *hold the head lower than the chest and hit between the shoulder blades.*

Recovery position

This is the position in which an unconscious person can breathe most easily.

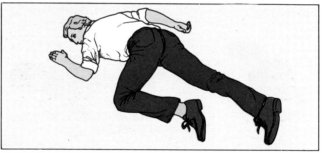

Turn the face to one side and bend the arm and leg on that same side. The other arm and leg should be straight. Continue to check pulse and breathing approximately every minute (see p.12).

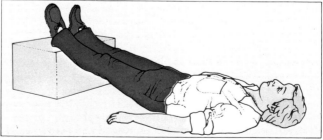

A conscious person recovers best from shock or from fainting by lying on the back with the feet raised. Keep the patient talking, to maintain consciousness.

Alphabetical directory of problems and treatments

Abdomen, burst
Lay the patient down. Do not touch the exposed intestine but cover it with a clean towel or smooth cloth. Do not give the patient anything to eat or drink. Summon an ambulance at once.

A burst abdomen is a rarity and occurs only very occasionally in people who have left the hospital after an abdominal operation or after a major injury, e.g. a knife wound or falling on a sharp edge of metal or glass.

Abdominal pain
Mild pain may be relieved by resting and taking tablets for indigestion. For severe pain, sit or lie in the most comfortable position. Pain in the lower abdomen is usually more serious than pain in the region of the stomach. If any severe pain continues for more than an hour, particularly with sweating, consult a doctor. See also A–Z: Abdominal pain.

Abrasion
This is a superficial injury to the skin, usually the result of a sliding fall, e.g. off a moving bicycle.

Examine the patient for other injuries. Treat *bleeding* (p.21) with firm pressure. If there are any small pieces of grit lying in the wound remove them with a pair of tweezers sterilized by boiling in water for five minutes. Wash the abrasion with soap and water, rinse thoroughly and dab dry. There is no need to cover the wound unless there is bleeding or it is likely to rub against the patient's clothing. If necessary cover with a dry sterile dressing, preferably with a non-adherent surface. Do not use ointments or creams. If the abrasion becomes infected or is deep and dirty it must be examined by a doctor and, if necessary, antitetanus injections given.

Accidental amputation
With a clean cloth apply direct pressure over the end of the stump, whether finger or limb, as hard as you can. Do not release pressure for at least twenty minutes. Call for an ambulance at once. Do not attempt to find a pressure point, or apply a tourniquet, unless you are trained in first aid.

If possible keep the amputated finger or limb. Put it into a clean plastic bag. Surround this with as much ice as possible and put it into a second plastic bag. It may be possible for a surgeon to stitch back the amputated part if the victim can be taken to a hospital within six hours.

Allergic reaction
Mild allergies usually appear as local skin reactions to contact with plants or chemicals. Apply a cold wet flannel or other cloth to the affected area, but do not scratch or rub it. Call a doctor if swelling develops.

A mild face or body rash may also be caused by an adverse reaction to a food or drug that has been swallowed. Lie down quietly, but call a doctor if the rash gets worse.

Severe allergic reactions (anaphylaxis) are usually caused by drugs but may also be due to an insect bite or sting. In these cases a highly irritating *rash* (p.40) covers the whole skin. The patient is also likely to suffer from breathlessness, collapse and shock. Place the patient in the *recovery position* (see p.18) and call a doctor, or take the patient to a hospital immediately. Ask if the patient has any emergency medication such as an inhaler for *asthma* (p.20) or antihistamine pills. If so, use as directed. Stay with the patient until help arrives. Observe pulse and breathing constantly as *heart massage* and *artificial respiration* (pp.13–17) may be required. See also A–Z: Allergy.

Angina   See *Heart attack*, p.36.

Asphyxiation
Remove the cause and give *mouth-to-mouth resuscitation* (p.15). Do not blow too hard.

Asthma attack
If the attack occurs indoors, the patient should sit on a chair with arms braced on a table. This allows the chest and arm muscles to be used to help breathing. Try to keep the back straight. If outdoors, the patient should use a fence or gate, or the shoulders of a friend, and rest his head on his

arms. The patient will know how to use a spray or tablets, if they can be found in a pocket or bag. If the symptoms do not improve after ten minutes, call for a doctor or take the patient to a hospital. See also A–Z: Asthma.

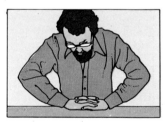

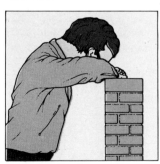

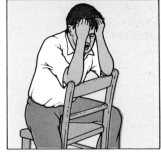

Asthma attacks *may be relieved if the arms are*   *braced to assist with breathing.*

Back injuries
If the person complains of severe backache, a fractured spine is a possibility. Do not move the patient if the injury

has been caused by a fall. Keep the patient warm by covering with blankets or a coat. Summon help at once. If the patient is not already lying down, place face-up on a hard, flat surface such as the floor. Examine the patient for *head injuries* (p.36) and possible *fractures* (p.29). Only if no help can be obtained should a person with a serious back injury be moved. This should be done only when the back has been completely immobilized with a long splint that stretches from above the head to below the bottom of the spine (see *Moving the patient*, p.38).

Bandaging   See *Fractures and bandaging*, pp.30–35.

Bites
Treat animal and human bites for *bleeding* (p.21) and clean the wound thoroughly by washing under cold water. When bleeding has ceased cover with a sterile dressing. All animal bites must be examined by a doctor or at a hospital as soon as possible as antibiotic treatment and a tetanus injection may be necessary. Antirabies injections may also be required for animal bites. See also *Insect bites*, p.37 and *Snakebite*, p.41.

Bleeding
Bleeding must be stopped as quickly as possible. Press hard with your fingers or hand with a clean handkerchief or cloth for 20 minutes. If it has not stopped, keep pressing for another 20 minutes.

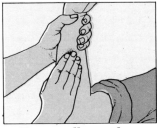

1. For a small wound, press hard with your fingers to stop the blood flow.

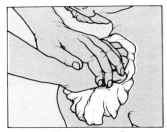

2. For a large wound, use a piece of clean cloth and press hard to stop bleeding.

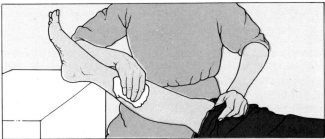

3. For varicose veins, which may bleed profusely if cut, raise the patient's leg and press on the site of the bleeding until professional medical assistance arrives.

In all cases, bleeding must be stopped as quickly as possible. This is best accomplished by pressing on the wound. If the broken blood vessels are closed by the pressure and the flow ceases, the natural clotting agents can be effective. After bleeding has stopped, clean the wound thoroughly and take the patient to a hospital for immunization against tetanus. Anyone who has suffered major bleeding will also be suffering from *shock* (p.41).

For a small wound, firm pressure with the fingers is usually sufficient. A large wound in which many vessels are damaged may require a clean cloth to be held against the hole so that all the damaged area is covered. A cloth is used for a large wound to allow pressure to be applied to a larger area, not to soak up the blood. For both small or large wounds, press on the wound as hard as possible for 20 minutes. Release the pressure after 20 minutes so that the rest of the circulation is not impaired. If the wound is still bleeding, press again for another 20 minutes.

Continuous bleeding from the mouth, ear, bladder or anus indicates an internal injury. Skilled medical treatment is required immediately. Lay the patient in the *recovery position* (p.18) and call an ambulance. Only if no ambulance can be called should other means be used to take the patient to a hospital. Minor bleeding from any of these places also requires medical attention.

Blister

A blister may be caused by a variety of injuries, e.g. *burns* (p.23), *allergic reaction* (p.19), or friction from shoes. Some infectious diseases, such as chickenpox or shingles (see A–Z for both), may also cause blisters.

Remove the cause, if still present, and wash the blister gently with some water. Do not puncture it, nor apply ointments, creams or lotions. Cover the blister with a light protective dressing till the fluid is naturally absorbed.

Breathing problems

Treat shortness of breath as an *asthma attack* (p.20). Rest, in a sitting position, improves the symptoms if the problem has nervous or emotional causes, but if breathlessness is severe or if it continues for more than 2 hours, consult a doctor. In an obvious emergency, call an ambulance or take the victim to a hospital at once. See also A–Z: Breathlessness.

Bruising

Bruising is due to bleeding into the tissues, which causes swelling and discoloration. It is usually caused by a physical injury, so make sure that there is no other damage, particularly to bones. If the swelling is accompanied by severe pain, take the patient to a hospital for further examination.

If there is no fracture, rest the area in an elevated position if possible or in a sling and apply a cold compress to reduce the swelling. Superficial bruises may also be caused by insect bites or by injections.

Burns and scalds
Fire. Immerse the patient immediately in cold water. If the fire is still burning or smoldering, wrap the patient tightly in a blanket or coat (note that synthetic materials, e.g. nylon, are dangerous in the presence of fire). Do not remove charred, burned clothes as these will be sterile.
Hot water. Immerse the patient immediately in cold water, removing the clothing as soon as possible. Keep the scalded area in cold water for ten minutes.
Chemical burns. Immerse immediately in cold water and remove the contaminated clothing as soon as possible. Continue bathing the damaged skin in cold water and soak for ten minutes. Do not rub the skin as this may cause further injury.

Cover the skin with a dry, sterile dressing. Do not use lotions or ointments. Large burns will rapidly cause *shock* (p.41). Deep burns, particularly those caused by electricity, and burns larger than 1cm ($\frac{1}{2}$in) – about the size of a postage stamp – are also dangerous. Take the patient to a hospital or, if he/she is shocked, call an ambulance at once.

Childbirth, emergency
1. Don't panic. Childbirth is a natural process.
2. Call a doctor or a midwife.
3. Sterilize equipment and wash hands thoroughly.
4. Do not hurry the mother. Let her set the pace.
5. Do not cut the umbilical cord. If medical help is delayed, the cord can be tied.

There is almost always more than half an hour from the time that the contractions of the first stage of labour start to the birth of the baby, so if labour begins, call a doctor or midwife or take the mother to a hospital as quickly as possible. If it is not possible to get to a hospital and professional help is unlikely to arrive in time, find somewhere warm, quiet and private, ideally a bedroom. Cover a bed, or an area of floor if there is no bed, with a waterproof sheet and a blanket or towel. Ask the mother to empty her bladder into a receptacle other than a toilet. She should then remove all the clothes below her waist and lie down comfortably on her side or on her back. Encourage her to relax between contractions and record their length and frequency. The cervix opens and the waters (amniotic fluid) may appear at this stage.

To assist the birth, you will need:
1. A blanket to wrap the baby.
2. Several towels.
3. Paper tissues, sanitary towels or clean cloths to be used as swabs.
4. Scissors and three 30cm (12in) pieces of string to tie the umbilical cord.
5. A saucepan or kettle of boiling water in which to sterilize string and scissors.
6. Clean water and soap to wash your own hands.
7. Antiseptic liquid.

Cleanliness is of utmost importance for the health of the baby and of the mother. Infection from your hands or from any of the accessories may prove fatal. Boil scissors and string for ten minutes, leaving them in the water until required, and wash your hands under running water for the same length of time.

The mother will feel the need to push down just before delivery. Rest between contractions is important at this stage. The mother should lie on her back and spread her legs apart as the contractions become stronger so that the first signs of the delivery can be seen.

When the baby's head is visible, rinse your hands in antiseptic liquid and cup them gently around the head. Do not pull on the head. As the head emerges ask the mother to stop pushing and to pant. This prevents the head from emerging too fast. Contractions may stop for a few minutes and the baby's head may rotate. Do nothing except support the baby's head.

When the shoulders appear, grasp the baby beneath the armpits and lift it up and onto the mother's abdomen. A newborn baby is slippery, so hold it firmly.

When the baby is completely delivered place it on the mother's abdomen with the head downwards to allow any mucus to drain from the mouth and nose. The baby's gasps and cries at this stage are normal and are the start of regular breathing. Wrap the baby in a blanket or towel and let the mother hold her child as soon as possible.

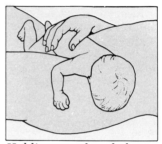

Holding a newborn baby.

Wait for the placenta (afterbirth) to be delivered. This appears as a mass of red fleshy tissue and is usually delivered within about 20 minutes after the birth of the baby.

Tie the umbilical cord with a piece of string about 15cm (6ins) from the baby's navel. **Do not** cut the cord unless you are sure that no medical help will arrive. If the cord must be cut, tie two more pieces of string tightly round it, one either side of the first piece. With sterilized scissors, cut between the two farthest pieces.

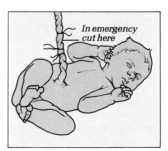

In emergency cut here

Tying the umbilical cord.

Complications

If the baby is born with the cord around the neck, loosen the cord and gently ease it over the baby's head.

If membranes cover the baby's face, they should be torn to

allow breathing. If the baby does not breathe after delivery, give *mouth-to-nose resuscitation* (see p.15).

If the baby's bottom or foot appears first instead of the head (breech delivery), do not interfere. Allow the birth to proceed normally, supporting the baby as required.

If contractions continue after the delivery of the baby and the placenta, a second baby may appear. The likelihood of twins is also indicated by the lump that remains in the abdomen after the first baby is born.

Bleeding after the birth may be due to part or all of the placenta being retained in the womb. Raise the foot of the bed and massage the mother's abdomen just below the navel. If the bleeding is heavy and does not stop within a few minutes, summon medical assistance urgently.

Children's emergencies
Many accidents occur to children because of inexperience and natural curiosity. In most cases the injury itself should be treated as if it had occurred to an adult. As a child may not be able to explain what has happened, it is of great importance to seek medical help or hospital treatment as soon as possible.

Remember, above all, that injured children need comfort and reassurance, that *shock* (p.41) develops more rapidly and is more serious in children than in adults, and that sweets, food or drink must not be given, because treatment in a hospital may require an anesthetic.

Coma   See *Unconsciousness*, p.43.

Concussion
A state of mental confusion that frequently follows a *head injury* (p.36). The person may not remember what has caused the mental confusion, nor have any recollection of what happened before the accident. Symptoms of headache, double vision and slurred speech are common. The patient must rest and be kept under constant observation in case of *unconsciousness* (p.43), which may occur sometimes. The patient should be kept warm, as *shock* (p.41) may commonly occur.

The symptoms of concussion will gradually improve, but it may be some days or weeks before there is complete recovery. Pain-killing drugs may be given for headache, but alcohol is prohibited. A doctor must be consulted.

Convulsions and fits
Do not try to restrict the movements of a person who is having convulsions. Move electric fires, furniture and other hard objects away from the person to avoid the danger of injury. When the fit has passed, leave the patient in the *recovery position* (p.18) to rest or sleep.

In babies and young children convulsions are often caused by a high *fever* (p.29). If convulsions occur, hold the child's head on one side and keep the air passage open so that the child can breathe. When convulsions stop, reduce the temperature by sponging the body with warm water. Call a doctor or take the child to a hospital immediately. See also A–Z: Convulsions and fits.

Cramp

An involuntary, painful muscle spasm that may affect the stomach or the extremities, particularly the legs and feet. The spasm is relieved by warming and massaging the affected part and often by stretching the muscles that are contracting. For example, to stretch the muscles of the thigh, calf or foot, try to straighten the leg with the toes raised and the heel pressed downwards. For cramp in the hand, pull the fingers firmly and steadily straight. Further cramps may be avoided by ensuring an adequate intake of fluids and salt. Consult a doctor if they persist. See also A–Z: Cramp.

Dehydration

This is indicated by thirst and lethargy, and by the skin appearing dry and slack. It is more common in hot weather or as a result of diarrhea, vomiting and fever. Treat initially by giving fluids to drink, but in small amounts such as a glassful at a time, in case vomiting occurs. Add a 5ml spoonful of salt and one of sugar to each 500ml (1 pint) of fluid. Too much fluid or fluid with too much salt may cause vomiting. If dehydration is associated with any other signs of illness, consult a doctor.

Dehydration occurs more quickly in children than in adults and can develop even faster in babies. The salt and sugar solution described above can be given, although sachets of sodium chloride and glucose oral powder, or similar proprietary preparations obtainable from your pharmacist, are more suitable for babies. If the child or baby is vomiting, with dehydration, a doctor should be consulted at once or the patient taken to a hospital.

Dental problems

Broken tooth. Place a piece of gauze over the jagged tooth and another inside the cheek to prevent its damaging the inside surface. Consult a dentist as soon as possible.

Gumboil. A painful swelling adjacent to a tooth from a dental infection. Take pain-killing drugs and antiseptic mouth washes, and consult a dentist as soon as possible.

Toothache. This may be due to a gumboil, dental decay or a broken tooth. Pain-killing drugs, combined with a cold compress on the side of the face, or drops of oil of cloves or alcohol applied directly to the painful tooth, may help. Consult a dentist promptly. See also A–Z: Toothache.

Ulcers in mouth. These may occur on their own or accompany a cold. They are white and painful. Treatment with sterile mouth washes and a variety of lozenges, obtainable from your pharmacist, will help until they heal naturally. If ulcers frequently occur, or remain for more than three weeks, consult your doctor or dentist. See also A–Z: Ulcer, mouth.

Diabetic emergencies

These are caused by an imbalance in the sugar levels in the blood. Either too much or too little sugar in the blood of a diabetic may lead to *unconsciousness* (coma) – see p.43.

Too much sugar, leading to a diabetic (hyperglycemic) coma, causes symptoms that include thirst, confusion, fever, vomiting, deep breathing and the gradual onset of coma.

Too little sugar in the blood, leading to a hypoglycemic coma, causes confusion, pallor and sweating. The coma develops rapidly.

If the person is conscious, give some sugar, in the form of lumps or sweets, because a little more sugar will not harm someone with an excess of blood sugar, whereas it will temporarily prevent a hypoglycemic coma. In both cases, call a doctor or take the patient to a hospital.

If the person is unconscious, place in the *recovery position* (p.18) and call an ambulance. Look for a medical identification card or disc round the patient's wrist or neck, in the pockets of the clothes or in any accompanying bags. Stay with the patient until help arrives. See also A–Z: Diabetes.

Dislocations

Treat all dislocations as if they were *fractures* (p.29). Support the affected joint in a sling or on pillows. Send for an ambulance or take the patient to a hospital. Anyone with a dislocation is likely to be suffering from *shock* (p.41). See also A–Z: Dislocation.

Drowning

Throw a life belt or buoyant object on a rope or, if necessary, swim with it to the drowning person. If needed give *mouth-to-mouth resuscitation* (p.15) at once, continue rescue and maintain artificial respiration afterwards. If occurring in ice **do not go onto ice unless securely attached** and you have additional help. Use a ladder if one is available and lie flat on the surface. See WINTER SPORTS: Accidents on ice, p.59.

Ear injuries

Bleeding from within the ear. This may be a serious sign, particularly if associated with a *head injury* (p.36). Consult a doctor at once. Bleeding from the external ear should be treated in the same way as any other form of *bleeding* (p.21).
Ear drum, burst. This may result from a *head injury* (p.36), or from flying while suffering from a cold or from sinusitis: the air pressure in the middle ear has been unable to equalize with the pressure within the plane, and this may have burst the ear drum. Severe pain precedes the bursting and may be followed by bleeding from the ear. Consult a doctor as soon as possible. Meanwhile do not put your head under water.
Foreign body in ear. Do not try to remove an object or insect from an ear as this may force it farther down and cause added injury. Take the person to a hospital at once.

Electric shock

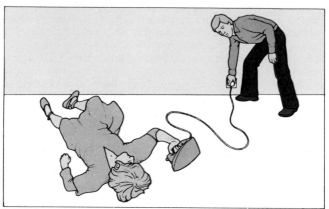

Electric shock. *Be sure to switch off the electricity at the circuit before touching the victim.*

Do not touch the victim. Switch off the appliance at the circuit or pull the plug out. If this is not possible use a wooden chair or broom to move the source of the electric current away from the victim. Resuscitate the victim with *heart massage* (p.13) and *artificial respiration* (pp.13–17). When the person is breathing normally, treat for *shock* (p.41). Take the person to a hospital for treatment of electrical *burns* (p.23) which may be invisible on the surface but extensive underneath.

Exposure   See *Hypothermia*, p.37.

Eye injuries
Major. Do not attempt treatment and do not try to remove any object stuck in the eye. Tell the patient to close both eyes, then place a clean handkerchief or dressing over the injured eye, which can be held in place by adhesive plaster or with a head bandage (see p.33 of *Fractures and bandaging*). Take the patient to a hospital at once.

Foreign body. It must be removed as soon as possible. Roll the eyelid up or down by pulling gently on the lashes. Wash the foreign body out with water or lift it out with a corner of clean material, e.g. a handkerchief. If there is continued discomfort take the patient to a hospital.

Chemicals. They must be rinsed out at once with cold water. Hold the head so the injured eye is on the lower side and wash it with running water. Cover the eye in the same way as when treating a major eye injury (see above). Take the patient to a hospital.

Black eye. This is caused by bleeding into the tissues, either from a direct blow to the eye socket or elsewhere on the head. Cover immediately with an ice pack or wet towel for at least ten minutes.

Fainting   See *Unconsciousness*, p.43.

Fever
By itself, it is seldom a major problem. However, *heat exhaustion* (p.36) and *heat stroke* (p.37) need immediate treatment. In severe illnesses the temperature is high and confusion is a common symptom. Sponging with tepid water will often help reduce the fever. A doctor must be consulted.

In young children, particularly infants, a high fever above 40°C (104°F) may be accompanied by *convulsions* (p.25), in which case sponging with tepid water will reduce the fever rapidly. However, a doctor must be consulted as soon as possible or the baby must be taken to a hospital. See CHART OF WHAT TO DO: Fever, p.94 and A–Z: Fever.

Fishhook injuries
Because a fishhook is barbed it cannot be withdrawn through the place at which it entered the skin. It must be pushed round until the barbed end emerges, then this must be cut off. The hook without the barb can be withdrawn easily. Consult a doctor as a tetanus immunization may be required.

Fit   See *Convulsions*, p.25

Food poisoning
It is usually due to a poisonous substance in food or to poisons produced by bacteria contaminating food. The onset of symptoms of severe vomiting, often accompanied by severe diarrhea, usually occurs within 2–4 hours of eating the meal. Some forms of food poisoning, which may be equally acute, are due to infection and the symptoms occur within 24–48 hours of the meal. Treatment for *dehydration* (p.26) and *vomiting* (p.44) must be given. In small children and babies a doctor should be consulted if severe symptoms last more than an hour. See also A–Z: Food poisoning.

Foot injuries
These are most commonly associated with fractures. In such cases, and if there is no bleeding, leave the shoe in place to act as a splint. See p.32 of *Fractures and bandaging*. If there is bleeding but no fracture, remove the shoe and sock or stocking carefully and treat for *bleeding* (p.21).

Fractures
A fracture may be suspected if there is unusual pain, swelling or deformity of any part of the body. If this has occurred you should treat the victim as you would for a fracture.

A fracture of the spine or neck is an extremely serious injury. Incorrect handling may permanently damage the spinal cord, producing paralysis. Signs of a fractured spine or neck will include severe local pain and sometimes loss of feeling or paralysis in limbs. Do not move the victim unless skilled help is available. The only time that a risk must be taken is if there is a life-threatening situation, e.g. fire or drowning.

As a general rule do not move the victim if there is any possibility that bones have been fractured – moving a fractured limb may cause internal damage. If a move is unavoidable, the fractured limb should be completely immobilized (see p.35 of *Fractures and bandaging* and *Moving the patient*, p.38).

Fractures in children are sometimes difficult to diagnose as the child may not complain of pain. If there is visible limping or an arm is not being used after an accident, the child must be taken to a doctor or hospital. See also A–Z: Fracture.

Fractures and bandaging

Any injury that may involve a broken bone or a dislocated joint should be treated as a fracture. Specific signs include pain that is made worse by movement, pain when the injury is pressed gently, swelling at the site of injury, and deformity of a joint or limb.

All fractures should be cleaned and covered if there is *bleeding* (p.21), supported with a sling or padded splint, and raised if possible to reduce swelling. The patient should be treated for *shock* (p.41). Bandaging is the first aid treatment for many types of fracture and the techniques used are described on pp.31–35.

Splints must be rigid. They must also be long enough and wide enough to prevent any movement once the injured part is bound firmly to them. Padding is used so that the hardness of the splint does not cause further damage to the limb. A leg splint is illustrated on p.35.

If the collarbone is fractured, it is important to hold the patient's shoulders back. To do this, tie a bandage round each shoulder by passing it under the armpit and tying it behind the shoulder. Use a third bandage to tie these two bandages firmly together, so that the shoulders are pulled backwards, and the broken ends of the collarbone prevented from damaging the lungs. Support the arm on the injured side in a sling.

If a rib is broken, support the arm on the injured side in a sling and take the patient to a hospital.

A crushed chest is particularly dangerous if there is a bubbling, gaping wound on the surface. Cover such a wound with a firm, clean bandage to prevent air from getting into the chest. Place the patient in the *recovery position* (p.18), lying with the injured side of the chest next to the ground so that the sound lung can breathe more easily. Call an ambulance so that the patient can be moved to a hospital on a stretcher.

Fractures that affect the skull, face or jaw require specialized attention. Make sure that the airway is not blocked by the injury (see *Clearing the airway*, p.13), and call an ambulance or take the patient to a hospital as soon as possible. See *Head injuries*, p.36.

Spinal fractures are indicated by severe local pain over the spine, and possibly weakness, loss of sensation or paralysis of a limb or another part of the body. The patient must not move or be moved because nerves or the spinal cord can be damaged. Call an ambulance if possible, and obtain the help of at least three other people. A stretcher is required, e.g. a large flat piece of wood, such as a door. Tie the patient's legs together at the thighs, knees and ankles. Carefully lift the patient onto the stretcher, preventing the body from moving, with one person holding the head, another the legs and the two others supporting the chest and pelvis. Tie the patient onto the stretcher until you reach hospital. See *Moving the patient*, p.38.

Bandaging is mainly used in the treatment of fractures. A bandage for support can be made from a belt, tie, scarf, or torn material. Most of the following illustrations show a bandage of the roll type, which can either be bought as a roll or made from a triangular piece of cloth.

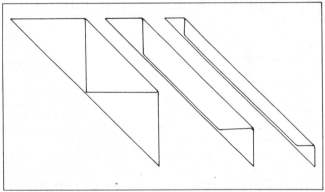

A triangular bandage can be made into a strip, as shown here. Begin by folding the triangle from the point to the longest side, then fold it in half, then lengthways, and finally in half again.

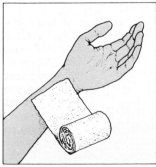

Start a bandage from the inside of a limb. Anchor the bandage with a double turn.

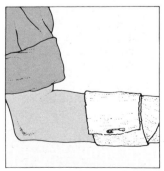

Finish a bandage on the outside of a limb, with the closure away from the body.

31

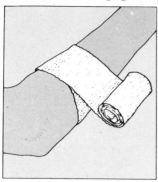

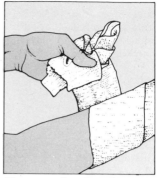

Wrap a bandage *with the roll on the outside. Overlap by about half the width.*

Unwrap a bandage *by gathering the loose cloth neatly into the hands.*

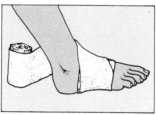

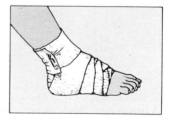

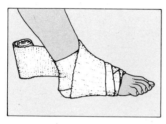

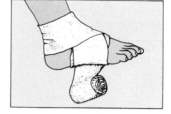

Foot and ankle bandages *are anchored underneath the foot. The bandage continues in a figure-of-eight pattern around the ankle, overlapping successive turns so that the foot is covered to below the instep and the ankle is supported. For an ankle bandage, finish on the outside, as illustrated. For a foot bandage, continue to the base of the toes and finish on top of the instep.*
Leg bandages *start at the ankle and continue up the leg to the knee. Use a second bandage if the first is short.*

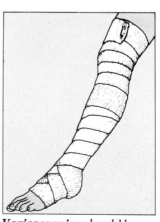

Varicose veins *should be bandaged spirally to give support to the leg.*

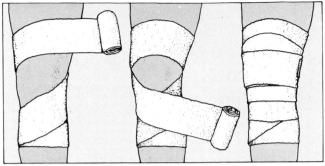

A knee bandage is anchored below the knee and bound in a figure-of-eight pattern passing behind the joint, crossing the kneecap and finishing on the outside.

Head injuries require bandaging if there is a wound that must be kept clean or if there is a dressing, for example one covering an eye or an ear, that must be held in place. A dressing should always be used with a head bandage.

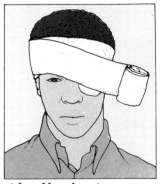

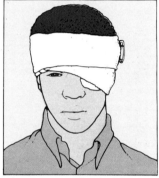

A head bandage is anchored round the largest part of the head. One turn drops lower than the others if it is required to hold a dressing in place. Further turns make the bandage secure. It fastens at the side.

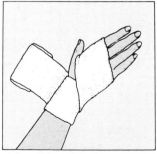

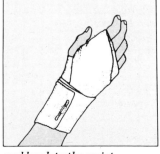

A hand bandage is anchored round the wrist, then passes over the back of the hand, across the palm and back to the wrist. Subsequent turns cover part of the fingers. The bandage finishes at the wrist.

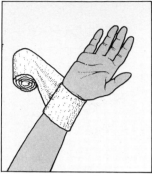

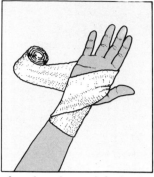

A wrist bandage is anchored round the wrist, then passed over the palm of the hand, in front of the thumb and round the back of the hand. This sequence is continued until the wrist is supported.

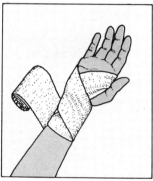

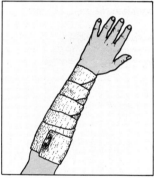

The bandage should be firm enough to prevent the wrist moving but should not affect the circulation to the fingers.

An arm bandage starts at the wrist and continues in a figure-of-eight pattern, as shown, to just below the elbow.

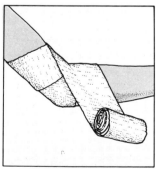

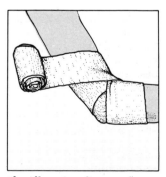

An elbow is bandaged like a knee. The bandage is anchored round the forearm, then passed round the elbow in a figure-of-eight pattern, crossing in front of the joint, and finally finishing on the upper arm.

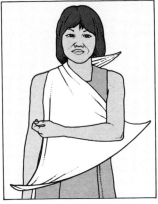

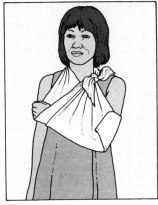

A sling *is made with a triangular bandage. The longest edge passes over the uninjured shoulder, beneath the injured arm,* *and is tied at the injured shoulder. The injured arm is raised and the point of the bandage is pinned for support.*

A sling is used to support an arm if the wrist or the forearm is injured, or if the arm requires support following the fracture of a rib or collarbone.

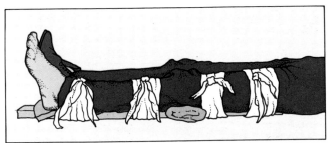

Immobilizing a limb. *A splint is required to prevent the limb moving. With the* *limb straight, tie a rigid support to the limb. Do not tie at the site of the injury.*

Frostbite
Frostbite is skin damage caused by cold stopping the circulation of blood. It usually affects extremities such as the toes, fingers and nose. Do not rub the affected part, and do not warm by putting in hot water. Warm a frostbitten hand by placing it in the armpit, or get into a sleeping bag. Loosen constricting clothing, drink something warm and get medical help as soon as possible. See *Hypothermia,* p.37.

Gunshot wounds
Gunshot injuries are characterized by small entry and large exit wounds. Treat as for severe *bleeding* (p.21). The victim suffers from shock and may also have serious internal injuries. Lay the victim on the floor in the *recovery position* (p.18) and call both an ambulance and the police at once.

Hair round a finger

This is particularly likely to occur in babies and young children who twist their fingers in their hair. The tight hair constricts the blood flow and this causes the finger to swell. Hair-removing cream or lotion must be used to dissolve the hair, before the finger becomes gangrenous. Visit a doctor or a hospital as soon as possible.

Head injuries

If the person is unconscious: Treat for *unconsciousness* (p.43).

If the person is conscious: Place the person in a comfortable position, either lying down or sitting in a chair, and treat for *concussion* (p.25).

Head wounds: Treat as for *bleeding* (p.21), using firm pressure over a clean piece of material for at least 20 minutes. Then use a head bandage (see p.33 of *Fractures and bandaging*).

All head injuries must be examined by a doctor. Any person who has been unconscious from a head injury must be taken to a hospital.

Heart attack

First *check the pulse* (p.12). If this has stopped, give *heart massage* (p.13). *Mouth-to-mouth resuscitation* (p.15) may also be required.

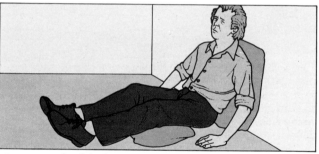

Heart attack. *If the heart is still beating the victim should sit in a comfortable position, ideally on the floor, with the back supported on pillows against a wall. This makes breathing as easy as possible. Stay with the patient until medical help arrives. Check the pulse regularly.*

If the person suffers a heart attack but the heart does not stop, the attack should be treated as angina pectoris. The main symptom is central chest pain, which typically occurs as a result of excitement or exertion. The pain of angina often spreads to the left arm and may also spread to the neck and abdomen. See A–Z: Angina pectoris and Heart attack.

Heat exhaustion

Symptoms include extreme fatigue, dizziness, fainting, sweating and cramp. They are caused by excessive loss of salts and water in sweat, and may occur following exertion in hot, humid conditions. Give fluid to drink in regular, moderate quantities – one cup at a time. Add a 5ml spoon of salt to every 500ml (1 pint) of fluid drunk. Consult a doctor in case further treatment is required. See *Dehydration*, p.26

Heat stroke
Symptoms include collapse, high temperature, hot, dry skin, confusion, and sometimes loss of consciousness. Treat for *heat exhaustion* (see p.36), immerse in cold water, and move the victim to a hospital as soon as possible.

Hemorrhoids
Also known as piles, they are dilated veins which may protrude from the anus (back passage). They may cause itching, or bleeding on defecation, and occasionally they thrombose, causing a painful, hard lump.

The itching may be relieved by soothing ointments obtainable from a pharmacist. A thrombosed pile may be relieved by applying a damp cloth with a plastic bag containing ice cubes (an **'ice pack'**) to the area. Pain-killing drugs will also help. See A–Z: Hemorrhoids.

Hernia (rupture)
Try to push the herniated bulge of tissue back into place and then consult a doctor. If the hernia is accompanied by local pain, swelling, general abdominal pain or vomiting, urgent medical attention is required as the hernia may cause intestinal obstruction. See also A–Z: Rupture.

Hiccups
A very common complaint that seldom lasts for long. There are a variety of treatments which include drinking from the wrong side of a cup, a sharp slap on the victim's back, and breathing into a paper bag for several minutes. Sometimes taking a deep breath and holding it for as long as possible is effective. See also A–Z: Hiccups.

Hypothermia (exposure)
A condition in which the body temperature is dangerously low. It is particularly likely to occur in babies and the elderly in cold weather.

Wrap the victim in blankets or coats, and give warm, sweet liquids to drink. Do not give alcohol or use a hot water bottle or an electric blanket because these cause blood to flow suddenly to the cold extremities and so cool the body temperature overall, which may kill the patient. Consult a doctor as soon as possible. See also SURVIVAL TECHNIQUES.

Insect bites and stings – See also *Stings*, p.42
Medical attention is not usually required unless the reaction to the bite affects more than the local area of the injury, or the insect is poisonous. Treat a local bite with anti-irritant (antihistamine) cream, or with cold water or an ice pack if nothing else is available.

Bees and ants have acidic venom, so apply a mild alkali such as sodium bicarbonate to the sting. The stings of wasps and hornets are alkaline, so a mild acid such as lemon or vinegar eases the pain.

Poisonous insects, such as certain spiders, scorpions and centipedes, are found in various parts of the world. If a person is bitten or stung by one of these, kill the insect and take it with the victim as quickly as possible to the nearest hospital or poison control centre. Fatalities from insect poisoning are rare, but immediate treatment is always necessary. For the most effective first aid treatment of an insect bite, see the treatment of *Snakebite*, p.41.

Ticks must be removed from the skin. Be careful not to leave the tick's head and jaws behind when its body is removed as this may lead to the bite becoming infected. Petroleum jelly, nail varnish, oil, alcohol or gasoline may help to make the tick loosen its jaws.

Labour, emergency   See *Childbirth, emergency*, p.23.

Migraine
As soon as the symptoms appear, drink three effervescent aspirin tablets in water. This form of aspirin is the most rapidly effective – even ordinary soluble aspirin may be absorbed too slowly. Lie down in a dark, quiet room as soon as possible. See also A–Z: Headache and Migraine.

Miscarriage
Signs of an impending miscarriage include backache, abdominal cramps, and vaginal bleeding during pregnancy. If these symptoms occur, a doctor should be called at once. The woman should lie down on a bed covered with a plastic sheet and towels. The best position is on the back with the knees apart and slightly raised. Additional towels placed between her legs are also helpful. It is important to keep the blood that comes from the vagina for the doctor to examine. Examination of the fetus may indicate the reason for the miscarriage. The fetus and afterbirth may not be noticed if the blood appears as a large clot. When bleeding ceases, replace the towels with a sanitary towel, but do not use tampons. See also A–Z: Miscarriage.

Mouth injuries
An injury that causes swelling may block the throat and lead to suffocation. Stings (see *Insect bites and stings*, p.37) and chemical *burns* (p.23) are most likely to cause swelling. To treat these, the patient should lie in the *recovery position* (p.18) and rinse the mouth repeatedly with cold water. Sucking an ice cube also helps. Take the patient to a hospital at once. For cuts in the mouth, apply direct pressure on both sides of the tongue or cheek. See *Bleeding*, p.21.

Moving the patient
Two people can move an immobilized person safely only with a stretcher. Otherwise a minimum of three people is required.

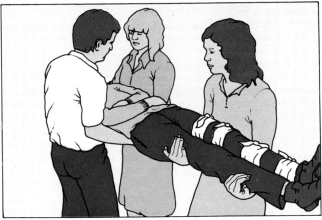

Three-person lift. *To move an immobilized patient, one person should support the shoulders and head, a second the hips, and a third the legs.*

Nosebleed

If the nose starts to bleed, sit with the head forward over a bowl so that the blood can drain from the nose. Breathe through the mouth. Press firmly on the soft lower sides of the nose to close the nostril for at least ten minutes. If this does not stop the nosebleed, lie flat on the back. An ice pack held over the bridge of the nose also helps. Old people with a nosebleed may feel faint, and it may be better for an older person to lie down with the head supported by several pillows, rather than to sit with the head over a bowl. When bleeding has stopped, rest for a further half-hour and avoid sniffing hard or blowing the nose for 48 hours. If bleeding occurs several times, or if it continues for more than half an hour, call a doctor. See also A–Z: Nosebleed.

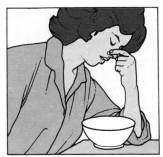

Nosebleed. *Pinch the nose and lean over a bowl. Breathe through the mouth.*

Nose injuries

Bleeding from the surface should be treated in the same way as *bleeding* (p.21) anywhere else on the body.

A broken nose is the result of a direct blow to the face and may be accompanied by a nosebleed or blockage of one nostril, deformity of the nose and black eyes. Apply an ice pack at once to reduce swelling and take the patient to a hospital. If correct treatment is given to the nose, deformity will be prevented, and an operation at a later date to break the nose again and straighten it will not be needed.

Piles *See Hemorrhoids, p.37*

Poisoning

In all cases, it is important to act fast. Call an ambulance and a doctor at once. In cases of gas poisoning, do not enter the room without proper breathing apparatus and skilled help.

If the person is unconscious, *check for breathing* (see p.12) and check for acid burns round the mouth. If the mouth is damaged and resuscitation is required, use the Holger Nielsen method (see *Artificial respiration, alternative methods*, p.16). Observe pulse and breathing until help arrives. Place in the *recovery position* (p.18).

If the person is conscious, ask the name of the poison. If strong acid or alkali has been swallowed, give water or milk to drink to dilute the poison. Place in the *recovery position* (p.18) and observe until help arrives.

If gasoline or cleaning fluid has been swallowed, it is better not to induce vomiting as this may cause further damage to the mouth and throat. Place in the *recovery position* (p.18) if the victim cannot walk.

For any other poisons, encourage vomiting by making the patient drink 500ml (1 pint) of water containing two large spoons of salt, or by giving a 5ml spoonful of ipecac syrup with a drink of water. Collect the vomit for analysis. Keep the patient awake by walking and talking.

Always take a person who has been poisoned to a hospital and always stay with the patient until help arrives. The hospital needs to know:

1. the name of the poison;
2. the time the poison was swallowed;
3. the time the patient was found;
4. whether the victim was conscious when found.

Also send any bottle or container near the patient, empty or half-full, and anything the patient has vomited.

Pulled muscle

Torn fibres within the muscle resulting from unexpected stretching or strain can cause a pulled muscle. It can be acutely painful and may sometimes resemble a fracture; if one is suspected, see *Fractures*, p.29

Treatment for a pulled muscle is rest, with pain-killing drugs and either a cold compress immediately after the injury or, some hours later, local heat in the form of an electric pad or a covered hot-water bottle.

Rash

In a child or a baby a rash may be a sign of over-heating, diaper rash, an allergy to certain clothing materials, soaps, chemicals, foods, plants or drugs, or it may indicate such illnesses as chickenpox, German measles (rubella), measles or scarlet fever. Determine the cause and remove it if possible. Consult a doctor if in any doubt or if other factors, such as fever, are involved. Cover the area to prevent scratching. A soothing lotion, such as calamine lotion, applied to the inflamed area may help to reduce the irritation. See also CHART OF WHAT TO DO: Rash, p.100 and A–Z: Rash.

Rescue from a height

The curiosity of an older child may lead to situations from which it is not easy to escape. Most commonly this occurs if the child climbs on a cliff or up a tree. When rescuing a child in such circumstances, it is most important to prevent panic. Do not show anxiety as this is likely to make the child frightened. Reassure the child and give advice about waiting in a secure position. Use a ladder to reach the child if possible. Otherwise call for skilled help, for example from the fire brigade or the coast guard. Keep talking calmly while waiting for help to arrive.

Ring stuck on a finger

This may occur after excessive use of the hand causes slight swelling of the tissues. Place the finger in ice, then cover it with grease and try to slip the ring off. If this does not work place a strong strip of thin plastic under the ring and over the knuckle. Gently try to pull the ring off. If the blood circulation is constricted and the finger begins to swell, go to a hospital at once.

Rupture   See *Hernia*, p.37.

Scalds   See *Burns and scalds*, p.23.

Scratches   See *Abrasion*, p.19.

Shock

The symptoms of shock are a pale skin, restlessness, confusion, anxiety, rapid pulse and shallow, rapid breathing. These symptoms are caused by the physical reaction of the body to a traumatic event such as an injury, heart attack, bleeding, burns, extreme or prolonged cold (exposure), or fear. The body reacts by reducing the blood supply to the skin, arms and legs so that an adequate supply to the vital organs (brain, heart and lungs) can be maintained. A person in shock should lie down, because this helps blood flow to the brain, and should be covered with blankets to reduce heat loss. Do not give extra warmth, alcohol, or hot drinks, as this dilates the skin's blood vessels and takes blood from the vital organs. Consciousness may fluctuate so try to keep the patient conscious by talking, and *check for breathing and pulse* (p.12) at all times. Keep the patient lying as still as possible and call a doctor or an ambulance. Stay with the patient until recovery from shock is complete. Anyone who is suffering from shock should be kept under medical observation for at least one hour.

Snakebite

Poisonous snakes are found in many countries of the world. The effects of their venoms vary from the mild poison of the adder or common viper found in most of the British Isles to the highly toxic venoms of the Indian krait, the African mamba or the American coral snake. Mild snake poisons may prove fatal in certain cases if the body reacts to them in an unusual manner; shock or heart attack are then more likely to cause death rather than the poison itself.

Identify the snake so that the correct antidote can be given. Kill it if possible and take it to the hospital with the victim. In all cases, the first treatment of snakebite must be to immobilize the bitten part. Take the victim to the nearest hospital or poison control centre as quickly as possible for the appropriate antivenom to be administered. Do not use a tourniquet, do not cut the wound, and do not allow the victim to walk if the bite is on the leg. Reassure the victim and treat for *shock* (p.41).

Splinter

If the splinter is small and the end protrudes from the skin, grasp it with a pair of tweezers and carefully pull it out in the direction opposite to which it entered the skin. Clean the splinter hole with antiseptic fluid. Do not attempt to remove a large splinter or one underneath the skin. Cover with a light dressing and consult a doctor. Deeply penetrating splinters, even if easy to extract, should be examined by a doctor as antitetanus injections may be needed.

Sprain

An injury to the ligaments and tissues of a joint, commonly the ankle or the wrist. Initially the best treatment for a sprain is to apply an ice pack or a cold compress to reduce the swelling. Then follow the directions for ankle and wrist bandages – see pp.32 and 34 of *Fractures and*

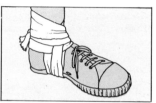

A sprained ankle can be supported temporarily by bandaging round the shoe.

bandaging. Rest the joint in a comfortable position. If in doubt, treat a sprain as a *fracture* (p.29).

Stab wounds

Do not move the weapon if it is still in place. Treat for *bleeding* (p.21), and stay with the victim, who will be suffering also from *shock* (p.41). Call an ambulance and the police immediately.

Stings – See also *Insect bites and stings*, p.37

Stings from plants or marine creatures such as jellyfish are painful and may cause extensive irritation of the skin. See *Allergic reaction*, p.19.

Plants may irritate the skin by injecting a poison, or by secreting a fluid, usually an oil, that is absorbed by the skin. Symptoms include itching, followed by the development of a rash and sometimes of blisters. Wash the affected area thoroughly with soap and water to remove all poison not yet absorbed. Do not touch any other part of the body, especially the face or eyes. If any skin irritation causes more than a minor, localized reaction, consult a doctor.

Jellyfish stings are often painful and may be dangerous if the shock prevents a swimmer from swimming properly. Wash the inflamed area thoroughly with alcohol, with vinegar added to it if possible, but do not use fresh water. Anyone stung by a Portuguese man-of-war should be examined by a doctor in case complications develop. For other jellyfish stings, medical treatment is required only if there is an allergic reaction or if the patient suffers from a medical condition such as a weak heart.

Stitch
A cramplike pain in the abdomen, usually occurring during exercise in those who are not fit. Lie the victim down and gently massage the abdomen. Do not exercise again for at least 15 minutes.

Sty
An infection around the root of an eyelash. Treat by tying an old handkerchief around a wooden spoon, dip into water as hot as you can stand, and apply the edge of the steaming handkerchief as a hot compress to the sty repeatedly for about ten minutes every 2–4 hours. This encourages the infection to discharge. Pain-killing drugs should be given if needed and a doctor consulted if the treatment is not effective within 24 hours.

Sunburn
For mild sunburn – sore and red skin, but without blisters – keep the affected areas covered, wear a hat and use sunburn lotions or oils to prevent the skin from drying out. For severe sunburn, marked by pain and blistering, treat as a *burn* (p.23); do not expose the skin to sunlight until it is completely recovered. Symptoms of *heat exhaustion* (p.36) may accompany severe sunburn. To obtain a tan without burning, start sunbathing for short periods only, in the morning and evening but not in the middle of the day.

Temperature See *Fever*, p.29.

Travel sickness
This is common in children over the age of two and tends to get better after puberty. It is likely to cause anxiety to both child and parents, and the advice of a doctor will prove valuable. Travel sickness pills, available from pharmacists, will help if taken before travelling, and will give confidence to the child. A damp sponge to wipe the mouth and face and plastic bags with wire tags to close them should be carried when travelling. See also A–Z: Travel sickness.

Unconsciousness
This most often occurs as a result of a *head injury* (p.36). If any possibility exists of a spine or skull fracture, **do not move the patient**: this may cause serious damage or death. Call a doctor or ambulance at once. *Check for breathing and pulse* (p.12), and that the *airway is clear* (p.13).

If the patient is breathing turn into the *recovery position* (p.18), then *check for breathing and pulse* (p.12) every minute. Look for any reason for loss of consciousness, e.g. a bottle of pills, evidence of a fall, or an identity bracelet or card indicating medical condition.

The chart below indicates courses of action to take.

If the person wakes normally:	1	Ask about possible reasons for unconsciousness. See also *Convulsions*, p.25.
	2	Ask the patient to move limbs to check for injury or paralysis.
If the person is drowsy, but can answer simple questions:	1	Try to keep the patient awake.
	2	Check for drug or alcohol abuse, *poisoning* (p.40) or *head injury* (p.36)
	3	Look for identity bracelet or card indicating medical conditions such as diabetes or epilepsy.
	4	Call an ambulance or doctor.
If the person does not wake:	1	Place in *recovery position* (p.18) and cover with a blanket.
	2	Call an ambulance or doctor.
	3	*Check for breathing and pulse* (p.12) until help arrives.

Urine, unable to pass (acute retention)
This may occur with cystitis or pregnancy, or in men with prostate problems. Take two pain-killing pills at once and lie in a hot bath for ten minutes. If this fails consult a doctor or go to a hospital. See also A–Z: Urine, retention of.

Vomiting
Help the victim to sit, kneel or lean in a comfortable position, with a bowl or plastic bag within reach. A spare bowl or bag is necessary if vomiting is frequent or copious. After an attack, the mouth should be rinsed with cold water. If an attack lasts longer than two hours, call a doctor. Beware of the danger of *dehydration* (p.26), particularly in babies and children.

If there is blood in the vomit or if the vomit appears black and granular, bleeding in the stomach is likely. Take the person to a hospital immediately. See also A–Z: Vomiting.

Winding
It results from a violent blow to the abdomen of the patient, who may gasp, collapse with *shock* (p.41), or occasionally become *unconscious* (p.43). Place in the *recovery position* (p.18) and loosen clothing around the neck and waist. Recovery commonly occurs within minutes but if symptoms of gasping and shock continue, medical advice must be sought at once or the patient taken to a hospital.

Zip-fastener injuries
These commonly involve the skin of the penis, particularly in children. The skin can be released by cutting the lower end of the zip, where the clip and material join, and opening the teeth from below.

HEALTH AND SAFETY

Introduction

In this section of the book the theme is: think ahead. Organize in advance for vacations, trips or sporting and physical activities. Take sensible precautions whether on the road or in looking after your own and your family's health. Positive preparation in all these areas is the key to a fuller, more enjoyable life.

Most of us find that going on vacation, particularly if it is abroad, is a time of excitement combined with anxiety. We feel excitement at the prospect of seeing new places, or even visiting ones we have enjoyed in the past; but we also feel natural anxiety about organizing the trip – what to take, the travelling details, passports, tickets, insurances, health requirements and so on. There are first aid and medical kits to think about, and the car, trailer and other equipment need to be checked for safety and good working order.

In the following pages, there is advice on FITNESS TO TRAVEL, KEEPING HEALTHY ON VACATION, and CAR SAFETY AND KIT. This is followed by ACCIDENT PROCEDURES, FITNESS TO DRIVE and SAFETY ON TWO WHEELS. These help you to prepare for a successful and safe trip, however long or short, whether in this country or abroad.

Health and safety are needed not only when travelling, but also in the home where sensible precautions can prevent accidents. DOMESTIC ACCIDENT PREVENTION points out 30 potential danger spots in the home and suggests practical remedies.

Good health too, like a smooth-running car, depends on care and preparation. A positive attitude to your own fitness will help prevent illness, and a sensible diet combined with exercise will maintain your well-being. GOOD HEALTH AND FITNESS offers much useful advice.

Unfortunately, illness may occur. The disabled and the elderly need help. Their comfort will depend on your knowledge of how to prepare and run a sickroom. This is essential in your own home, but unfortunately it can sometimes also be necessary on vacation if unexpected illness afflicts a member of your party. At such times, your skill may prevent further complications – CARE OF THE SICK AT HOME provides invaluable guidance, including advice on the problems of old age and the care of an elderly patient.

Many people on vacation undertake physical activity for which they may not be fully prepared. Winter and summer sports need fitness and skill. CAMPING, HIKING, WINTER SPORTS and WATER SPORTS assist you in ensuring enjoyment with safety.

Yet even the best-prepared plans can go wrong. An accident may leave you exposed and in danger. SURVIVAL TECHNIQUES will help you stay alive and prevent you from increasing your danger by taking the wrong course of action.

Fitness to travel

Before you leave make sure that you are fit to travel. If you have any health problems consult your doctor. It is not advisable to travel with a fever as it may develop into something more serious by the time you arrive. If you have a cold, an ear or sinus problem, the pressure differences of flying may cause pain and even a perforated ear drum.

Those planning to take part in physical sports such as mountain climbing, scuba diving, or air sports such as hang gliding and sky diving, are well advised to have a comprehensive medical check-up before departure, as many clubs organizing these sports demand a medical certificate of physical fitness. Those with chronic disorders or physical handicaps (such as diabetes mellitus, heart, lung or arthritic problems) or neurological problems (such as epilepsy or after a stroke) should consult their doctor. Anyone who has recently had a major operation, heart attack, colostomy, asthma or psychiatric disorder, should ensure that he or she is medically fit to travel.

Sea travel

Seasickness may be prevented by taking antinauseant pills the night before, another pill two hours before departure and one pill every 4–6 hours on the voyage. As these may cause drowsiness it is advisable not to drive a car immediately after a short crossing. On longer voyages the ship's doctor should be informed if a person is taking regular medication and is seasick, so that appropriate treatment can be given before dehydration occurs.

Air travel

Women in the last two months of pregnancy must inform the airline; many companies will refuse to accept them, so be sure to check beforehand. Jet lag is frequently a problem after arrival, but sedative drugs, which can be prescribed by your doctor, may help to obtain good sleep over the first few days. During the flight, light meals are preferable to large ones. It is also important to remember that dehydration may occur on long flights, so drink plenty of fluid, although alcohol should be avoided. Loose-fitting clothing and shoes will make the flight more comfortable – feet particularly tend to swell so that tight shoes are often difficult to put on again.

Be sure to remember that all regular medication must be taken on the time basis of your country of departure: do not change to a new time zone until after you arrive.

Car and inland travel

Particularly for children, travel sickness is a common problem in cars and buses, although it is less frequent on trains. The antinauseant regime suggested for sea travel may prevent this occurring. In hot climates ensure that there is plenty of fluid to drink and that old people exercise whenever they get out of the vehicle, to prevent excessive stiffness.

Returning home
The journey home may be every bit as fatiguing as the outward one. It is therefore important to allow sufficient time for an adequate night's sleep, following a light meal, on returning home.

Some illnesses, particularly tropical ones, may take some time to develop, so if you become ill be sure to tell your doctor that you have recently been abroad.

Keeping healthy on vacation

When going on vacation, and particularly when travelling abroad, certain precautions will help to ensure that problems of ill health do not arise, or that, if they do, they are prevented from becoming serious. See also COUNTRY-BY-COUNTRY MEDICAL AND MOTORING REQUIREMENTS, p.184.

Checklist – Recommended immunizations for travellers

Immunization	Schedule and protection
Cholera	International Certificate valid for six months beginning six days after one injection. *All Asian countries; Australasia; many African countries.*
Gamma globulin (immune serum globulin)	One injection just prior to departure. Gives three to four months' partial protection against infectious hepatitis. *Countries outside northwestern Europe, USA, Canada and Australasia where sanitation is of a low standard.*
Poliomyelitis	Three doses of oral vaccine at four- to six-week intervals. Valid for five years. *All countries.*
Tetanus	Three injections: the second, one month after the first; the third, six months later. Valid for five years, and often combined with the typhoid immunization. *All countries.*
Typhoid	Two injections two to four weeks apart. Gives up to two years' partial protection. *As gamma globulin (excluding Australasia).*
Typhus	Two injections seven to ten days apart. Valid for one year. *Southeastern Asia; India; Ethiopia.*
Yellow fever	International Certificate valid for ten years beginning ten days after one injection. *Some central African countries; some South American countries.*

All immunizations should be at the discretion of your own doctor.

Checklist – Drugs for travelling abroad

N.B. If you are travelling in a region where malaria is endemic you must take antimalarial drugs such as chloraquine or Daraprim. The course should be started before you leave and continued throughout your visit, and should be kept up for **at least** one month after your return.

General
1. First aid kit (see pp.8–9)
2. Clinical thermometer
3. Sunburn cream or lotion
4. Insect repellant cream
5. Water-sterilizing tablets
6. Travel sickness pills
7. Salt tablets
8. Aspirin tablets (300mg: one bottle) – for fever and pain
9. Loperamide capsules (2mg: 20) – for diarrhea
10. Antihistamine tablets (one bottle) – for insect bites and colds

For children and infants
1. Loperamide syrup (100ml: from your doctor) – for diarrhea – or kaolin mixture (100ml) – for infants
2. Infalyte – premeasured packet – for diarrhea and vomiting
3. Acetaminophen mixture (100ml) – for fever and pain

Remember also
1. Drugs taken on a regular basis by any member of your party
2. Additional drugs, e.g. sleeping pills or antibiotics, recommended by your doctor

General advice

Take out sufficient health insurance to cover the possibility of hospitalization. Some insurances cover the cost of repatriation as well as all incidental expenses for your family in the event of an emergency. If you suffer from any recurrent or permanent medical problem, or if you are taking a young child abroad, discuss specific precautions with your doctor before you depart and ensure that you pack adequate supplies of all drugs that are being taken on a regular basis. A phrase book giving foreign names of illnesses and symptoms may come in useful.

Take great care when sunbathing until you are fully acclimatized. At first, lie in the sun for only ten minutes in the morning and ten minutes in the late afternoon. Increase this by ten minutes a day until you are tanned but not burned. Never lie in the sun during the hottest part of the day, and remember that children can get sunburned just as easily as adults. Ensure that all members of your party always use a suntan lotion.

Avoid unwashed food, cooked foods that have been allowed to cool without refrigeration and unsterilized water, as any of these may carry infectious organisms that can cause food poisoning. Do not swim within two hours of eating a large meal, as this can lead to muscle cramps.

Car safety and kit

Car manufacturers are acutely aware of safety factors when designing new models. In most cars the central compartment containing the driver and passengers is designed as a rigid structure so that the hood and trunk will 'crumple' easily in an accident, thus acting as a shock absorber protecting the central compartment. More and more cars are using shatterproof glass in the windshield, instead of tempered glass, as an additional feature. Most cars will now have child-proof locks on rear doors, thus ensuring that the door can be opened only from the outside when the lock is engaged.

The driver and front-seat passenger should always wear seat belts, except when reversing. Certain modifications may be made for medical reasons but there are few, if any, medical reasons why someone should not wear a seat belt. Babies or children under the age of two should never travel in the front seat, and provision should be made for children under the age of ten to be properly supported when wearing a seat belt. Some cars, usually more expensive models, have rear-seat belts, which should be worn by passengers at all times.

Specially designed seats and seat belts are available for use by babies and children and should be fitted in cars where a member of the family falls into this age group. These not only protect the child in the event of an accident but also stop them from distracting the driver by reaching for the controls. Dogs should travel on the back seat, or, in station wagons, behind a fitted grid.

Below is a suggested checklist of safety precautions to take both for everyday and long trips. Every motorist, of course, will have different ideas, but these are basic essentials that promote safety when driving. For various requirements when travelling abroad, see also COUNTRY-BY-COUNTRY MEDICAL AND MOTORING REQUIREMENTS, p.184.

Checklist – Before long journeys and vacations

1. Check spare tire.
2. Check water in cooling system; add antifreeze in winter.
3. Check windshield washing tank. Add antismear fluid; treble quantity in winter to prevent freezing.
4. Check windshield wipers are working. Replace worn blades.
5. Check alignment of headlights.
6. Check wheel jack and brace are in position.
7. Fit fire extinguisher.
8. Check contents of first aid kit (see pp.8–9).
9. Before leaving, wash and wax car to give protection against sun, salt or winter weather.
10. Put in trunk:
    spare fanbelt, jump cables, spare bulbs, toolbox, towrope, tire pump.
    In severe winter conditions:
    waterproof clothing, extra coats, boots, solid-fuel burner and food, matches, flares, snow chains.

continued on next page

---

11. Put in car in a secure place:

auto club membership card and handbook (if you have it);
first aid kit;
this book;
driver's license and insurance documents;
blanket;
'iron rations', e.g. nuts, biscuits, sweets;

paper tissues;
maps and route plan;
plastic bags with ties, for rubbish and vomit;
plastic water container, full, with mugs;
sunglasses;
toys for children;
tire pressure gauge;
'wipes' for dirty hands.

Checklist – Before travel abroad

1. Consult your auto club about the country or countries you are planning to visit.
2. Take advice about 'masking' headlights when driving on opposite side of road to that for which your car is designed. (This is a legal requirement.)
3. Obtain a reflecting red triangle. (This too is a legal requirement. In some countries two are required.)
4. Carry a spare-part kit from manufacturers of your car.
5. Check car insurance policy and make sure your are covered for personal liability as well as for any damage to the car.
6. Check validity of US driver's license in countries you intend to visit, or obtain international driving permit.
7. Check personal and health insurance for cover abroad, and immunization requirements.
8. In some countries a first aid kit is legally required to be carried by all cars.
9. Get maps, guidebooks and route plans.
10. Get a continental handbook.
11. Have foreign dictionaries and phrase books.

Checklist – Before each day's driving

1. Listen for weather and road forecasts on radio.
2. Check gasoline.
3. Check oil and water.
4. Check front and rear lights, brake, backup and number-plate lights.
5. Check tire pressures and depth of tread, including spare, and adjust (if recommended by manufacturer) for increased load or highway driving. N.B. Remember to reduce pressure again when carrying normal load.
6. Clean windshield, rear window and rear-view mirrors.
7. Realign rear-view mirrors if necessary.

Checklist – On getting into car

1. Check brakes are working.
2. Check horn is working.
3. Check driver and front-seat passenger are wearing seat belts. Rear-seat passengers should wear them, if available, and small children and babies should be securely strapped in child seats.

Accident procedures

If you are involved in an accident while driving a road vehicle there are certain laws that you **must** obey. These are summarized in the first two checklists below.

An accident is defined thus:

1. When someone other than yourself is injured;
2. When you have damaged another vehicle;
3. When you have injured an animal, other than one in your own vehicle (an animal is legally defined as a horse, ass, mule, cow, sheep, pig, goat or dog);
4. When you have damaged someone else's property.

If you have caused or have been involved in an accident, carry out the procedures in the following checklist (these will vary somewhat from state to state).

Checklist – At a road accident

1. Stop and stay at the scene for a reasonable time even if no one else is present. (Remember how long you stayed.)
2. Give your name and address, as well as that of the owner of the vehicle if you do not own it, and the vehicle's registration number to anyone who has good reason to ask for them, e.g. the owner of the other car involved in the accident, or the owner of the injured animal or damaged property.
3. Obtain the name and address of the other person to whom you have given your name etc. If they do not own the other vehicle, or the injured animal or damaged property, ask for the name and address of the owner and the registration number of the other vehicle.
4. If it is not possible to give your name etc. to the other person (e.g. if no one else is present when you have the accident) you **must** report it to your insurance carrier as soon as you can and, in any case, within 24 hours.

If you have, in addition, injured someone, carry out the procedures in the following checklist.

Checklist – For injury at a road accident

1. Your first priority should be to call for an ambulance, if necessary, and the police.
2. Produce your own certificate of insurance and ask the other driver for his license, registration and certificate of insurance.
3. Exchange names, addresses, registration numbers and insurance I.D. numbers. As soon as possible, report the accident, along with a description of the damage or injury, to your insurance carrier.

In addition to your legal obligations you also have to inform your insurance company and fill in the claim form that will be sent to you. The nearest office of your auto club, such as the AAA, may be able to help you with any questions by connecting you with its insurance agents.

You will therefore need the following information.

Checklist – For insurance claim
1. The name and address of the other driver, injured person, or owner of the property or animal.
2. The name and address of the owner of your vehicle, injured animal or damaged property if different from your own.
3. The names and addresses of all witnesses – both those in the vehicles and those independent of the accident.
4. A detailed description of any injury to yourself and anyone else.
5. A detailed description of damage to vehicles, property or animals.
6. The name and address of the other driver's insurance company and the number of the certificate of insurance, if it is produced.
7. The other vehicle's make, model, year and registration number.
8. The number (on the shoulder) of any policeman present.
9. The number of the other driver's license or international driving permit.
10. The time and date of the accident.
11. The approximate speed of the vehicle(s).
12. The condition of the road surface, its width, markings and road signs.
13. Weather conditions and light conditions, e.g. rain, dusk, and whether there were any street or vehicle lights.
14. Any marks or debris from the accident on the road surface.
15. The manner in which the other vehicle was being driven.
16. Whether the driver and passengers were wearing seat belts.
17. A sketch map of the scene of the accident, showing the direction in which the vehicles were travelling, the point of contact and where they stopped after the accident. A sketch map is also necessary to show the position on the road of any animal when it was injured.
18. If a camera is available, take photographs of the accident.

Fitness to drive

Applicants for a driver's license have to state that they are medically fit to drive a car and that if at any point in the future they become unfit they will inform the local Department of Motor Vehicles. Certain medical conditions, such as epilepsy, partial paralysis or mental illness, make the applicant, in general terms, unfit to drive. However, many such people may be able to obtain a driver's license with a suitable modification to their car and by reporting the applicable restrictions to their local licensing bureau. It is unnecessary to inform the Department of Motor Vehicles about a temporary disability, such as an arm in a cast, lasting less than three months. If, however, the disability should last longer than this, or should a new disorder such as epilepsy develop, the Department of Motor Vehicles must be informed. If you have any problems about deciding what to do, discuss this with your doctor.

You should also inform your insurance company about any change in your health that may affect your ability to drive. After the age of 70, your insurance company may require an annual medical examination and a certificate signed by your doctor, before renewing your policy. At any age, you are required to have regular eye examinations.

Alcohol and Drugs

It is an offense to drive or to be in charge of a vehicle while under the influence of alcohol or drugs.

Alcohol is well known to affect driving ability and it is an offense to drive with alcohol levels above a legally defined level. Each state has its own laws, but dangerous levels are as follows: in breath 35 micrograms per 100ml, in blood 80 milligrams per 100ml, and in urine 107 milligrams per 100ml. A convicted person can lose his or her driver's license. In addition, some states may impose much harsher penalties, such as jail sentences, for repeated drunk driving offenses.

There is no clear-cut definition of 'unfitness to drive' due to drugs. However, many drugs, whether prescribed by a doctor or obtained over the counter from a pharmacist, may slow down reactions. Any of these drugs may have their sedative effect greatly increased by small amounts of alcohol or fatigue. Sometimes the bottle will be marked with a warning about the sedative effect of the drug.

Fortunately for most people these problems do not apply. The most important thing is to remain relaxed and alert while at the wheel and to avoid undue fatigue, heavy meals or even small amounts of alcohol before driving. Make sure also that your seat is properly adjusted and comfortable, that the ventilation system maintains a flow of fresh air and that distractions from within the car – such as noisy children or argumentative passengers – do not occur. If you find your concentration fading or feel tired, stop, get out, and do some simple exercises to relax your muscles. It is a good idea to have something to eat and drink before driving again.

Safety on two wheels

Motorcyclists and bicyclists have a high accident rate. Their cycles are less visible to drivers of other vehicles and give little or no protection if they are involved in an accident. All cyclists therefore should wear clothing that is not only protective but contains also Day-Glo and reflective material so that they are conspicuous both by day and night.

Motorcyclists

Both driver and passenger are legally required to wear crash helmets. There is a great variety of helmets from which to choose, but be sure your helmet has the US Department of Transportation (DOT) stamp of approval. It is essential to have a helmet that fits properly, whether it is an open-face or full-face type, with straps that are easy to adjust and comfortable to wear. Eye protection is also required: either a visor or goggles.

If a visor is worn – and most crash helmets now have them fitted – it is important to remember to pull it down when riding, as it can pull the helmet backwards if not in place. The visor should be replaced if it becomes scratched. Most helmets will become damaged after one hard knock. If this happens, even if the helmet appears intact, it should be replaced immediately, as it may shatter in a further accident, which could prove fatal. Wash the helmet with water, and do not let it come into contact with gasoline or other chemicals, or with Scotch tape or decals, as these damage the helmet fabric. Since most helmets become damaged by repeated small blows, it is sensible to replace them after three years' use.

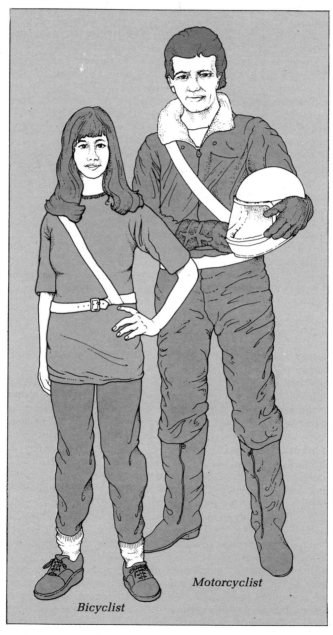

Motorcyclist

Bicyclist

Motorcyclists should also obtain properly designed protective clothing that is not only warm but also capable of keeping the rain out. Well-fitting boots with protective metal toecaps and soles will be an additional safety factor.

Motorcycles vary greatly in size and speed. Learner riders must obey all of the highway speed and passing regulations. It is important to develop and improve driving techniques, but this can only be done with skilled instruction and by practicing on quiet roads. It is also essential to know how to cope with an unexpected skid, and at all times to remember that other road users may not be able to see you, even if you have your headlight on. For a safe career on two wheels, drive sensibly at all times and take great care in all road and traffic conditions.

Bicyclists

A bicycle is much easier to ride than a motorcycle, but nevertheless your machine should be of the right size, with handles and seat adjusted to your height: when you are seated the toes of both feet should be able to touch the ground on either side. Keep your machine well-maintained and pay particular attention to the tires and brakes. Remember that skirts and scarves can easily be caught in the spokes. Bottoms of trousers should be held in place by bicycle clips or tucked into socks. You should wear Day-Glo and reflective material on your clothes, and additional strips can also be fixed to the pedals, spokes and rear of the bicycle. At night you must have a fully-working front and rear light. Take particular care at pedestrian crossings, and when passing parked cars remember that a door may be carelessly opened.

Camping

Many people enjoy camping and trailer vacations, not only because they are cheaper than hotels but because they also allow freedom and flexibility in choosing where to stay that will be particularly appreciated by families with young children. Even if you do not have your own trailer or camping equipment it is possible to rent everything that you need for a mobile vacation. However, it is important to plan and complete arrangements early in the year, as equipment and recreational vehicles will be booked early for the peak vacation times. Experience of previous vacations is not important but it is essential to take advice and plan ahead. If you are going abroad you should familiarize yourself with the regulations of any countries through which you will be passing.

When towing a camper or trailer it is essential to have a car that is adequately powered for the weight that it is pulling, to have the correct type of towbar fitted by your garage, and to have extended wing-mirrors or a special kind of rear-view periscope mirror that enables you to look through the windows of your trailer to the road behind. You cannot exceed 50mph or use the fast (passing) lane on highways. It is difficult to judge distances and angles when reversing a trailer or camper, and anyone lacking experience should practice on a quiet road with help from at least one other member of the party.

Your local Automobile Association and *Woodall's Campground Directory* can provide excellent and essential advice, including a list of approved sites throughout the United States.

Hygiene

Cramped conditions and lack of facilities are no excuse for lowered standards of hygiene. A fully organized camp and trailer site may nevertheless have a low standard of hygiene, and food poisoning can occur unless common-sense precautions are taken. Hands must always be washed before preparing food, especially for babies, and cups, plates and cutlery should be washed after every meal. Refuse should be disposed of in sealed plastic bags, and empty cans and glass wrapped in paper before putting in covered bins. Piped water in the US, Britain and Northern Europe is usually safe but farther south it is advisable either to boil it or to use water-sterilizing tablets. Any water taken from streams, however clear and apparently clean, must be assumed to be contaminated.

On many campsites toilet and washing facilities are excellent, but if you use your own it should be emptied daily and disinfected before further use.

Equipment and clothing

There is an immense variety of equipment available, ranging from recreational vehicles of a specification so high that they have central heating and hot running water, to the other extreme – the simple tent, groundsheet and sleeping bag. Whatever your choice of accommodations, it is essential to have adequate cooking facilities. In a trailer, cooking is usually by bottled gas which must always be turned off after use. With a tent, solid fuel stoves are easy and safe to use. It is important, however, that your stove should be erected on level and firm ground, for a fire at a campsite is extremely dangerous. Anyone going on a camping vacation should be sure to take a small, hand-held fire extinguisher.

Clothing will depend on how much you can store and on the type of climate you expect to encounter. Several layers of light clothing will keep you warmer than one heavier garment. A lightweight waterproof garment for each member of the party is essential, for rain can ruin a vacation if everyone gets soaked and there are no facilities for drying clothes.

Food

Canned food will keep well, and, as many trailers have small refrigerators run off the gas, fresh food is also easy to store. Insulated food containers will help to keep food fresh for 24 hours in hot climates. Any food that appears to be going bad should be thrown away at once.

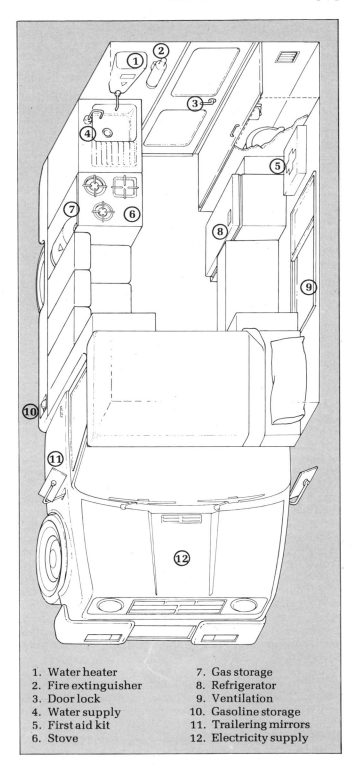

1. Water heater
2. Fire extinguisher
3. Door lock
4. Water supply
5. First aid kit
6. Stove
7. Gas storage
8. Refrigerator
9. Ventilation
10. Gasoline storage
11. Trailering mirrors
12. Electricity supply

Hiking

Preparation

Hiking involves more than simply a country walk. Plan the route carefully using maps and guidebooks and never set out on a hike alone if it is going to take you far from help. If you plan to go on a walk lasting more than five hours, always take at least two companions. Before you leave tell someone where you intend to go and the estimated time you hope to arrive at your destination; keep to your planned route and let this person know when you have arrived.

It is important that the hike should be within the capabilities of the least experienced member of the party. Before leaving, listen to the weather forecast and be prepared to cancel your plans if there is any likelihood of danger (for example from fog or snow). This is particularly important when hiking in mountain districts, where local weather forecasts may be posted at the beginning of commonly used paths. Finally, make sure that your planned hike can be finished within daylight hours, estimating the rate of walking as that of the slowest member of the party.

While hiking it is better to have frequent small meals and small amounts of drink than to try to walk with an overfull stomach.

Accidents

It is crucial to give the proper first aid treatment quickly to prevent the onset of shock (see FIRST AID, p.41) after a minor accident, particularly in cold conditions when prompt action will reduce the chances of hypothermia. In an emergency, fear can be a major factor in increasing danger. Companions of an injured or ill person, for example, may find their assessment of a situation unfavourably altered by their anxiety. It is therefore important to pause, consider the situation and balance the risks before making a decision about what to do.

Often it is safer to find a secure, sheltered spot for the victim than to try to move an injured person in dangerous conditions. One person must stay with the victim, who should be placed on plastic waterproof clothing to give protection from the cold ground. Rucksacks, branches and clothing can act as a screen for additional protection. Hypothermia (see FIRST AID, p.37) is caused by a combination of factors, including fatigue, hunger, cold, high winds and injury. This can happen to the young and fit as well as to the old, particularly in wintry conditions on mountains. See SURVIVAL TECHNIQUES, pp.61–65.

A waterproof backpack is vital, with a frame that fits easily on the back of the person carrying it. It should be adjusted for comfort before starting the hike. Put in essentials before the luxuries, and next to the frame carry sufficient spare clothing to meet any weather conditions. The minimum contents which should enable you to meet most contingencies are as follows.

Checklist – Backpack survival kit
1. Map and compass
2. Signalling device, e.g. whistle or metal mirror
3. Matches or lighter
4. Nylon rope
5. First aid kit contents:

one elastic adhesive bandage (5cm wide);	safety pins (3);
small Band-Aids for cuts;	antiseptic cream;
	antidiarrheal medication;
	aspirin tablets (300mg);
triangular bandage;	antihistamine tablets;
lip salve;	water-sterilizing tablets

6. Water, sufficient for hike
7. 'Iron rations', e.g. chocolate, biscuits, nuts, sweets, dextrose tablets (salt tablets in hot weather)
8. Flashlight and spare battery
9. Waterproof and warm clothing, gloves etc.
10. Sunburn cream

Winter sports

Skiing

Whatever your standard, you should be properly clothed and equipped. Before going on a skiing vacation check your own clothing and equipment and rent any other essentials. Your hat and gloves must be warm and well-fitting. Goggles cut out glare from the side and provide better protection for the eyes than sunglasses. Brightly coloured jacket and trousers made of water-resistant, lightweight material are easy to identify in the event of an accident. Release-bindings on the skis are essential and should be checked daily.

Start a program of increasing exercise at least two months before departure to achieve good physical condition by the time you arrive. Do not try to be over-ambitious: join a class matched to your basic level of skill.

Ice

The temptation to walk or skate on ice before it is thick enough is understandable but very dangerous. Safe ice is usually found on ponds and small lakes, and sometimes on streams with a sluggish flow. It is always thinner at the edges or under overhanging trees, bridges and banks. Ice on tidal waters and on fast-flowing rivers breaks easily, even though it may be thick, due to the frequent changes in stress.

All skaters must learn how to fall on ice by relaxing and letting the fall take its natural course. Leaning forward with an outstretched hand at the beginning of the fall will allow the arm and body to slide along while the elbow absorbs the jolt.

Accidents on ice

If you fall through the ice, do not panic, and **do not** attempt to climb out. Kick your feet to the surface behind and extend your hands and arms onto the surrounding ice. Swim forward, breaking the ice in front of you, until firmer ice is reached and you can wriggle onto it. Do not stand up until you are absolutely sure that you are on solid ice.

A more common form of accident is to trip and fall on the ice, cracking but not breaking through it. **Do not** stand up: this will cause the ice to break into a hole. Lie across the ice and wriggle or roll away from the cracked area. Do not stand up until you are sure the ice is firm enough.

Anyone who has fallen through or onto the ice must change clothing as soon as possible to prevent hypothermia (see FIRST AID, p.37). For further advice on rescuing a victim from ice, see Drowning (FIRST AID, p.27)

Water sports

If you intend to take part in water sports you must be able to swim well enough to do so in wet clothing.

Swimming
All members of the family should learn to swim as early as possible. However, no one should swim within two hours of eating a large meal, after drinking alcohol or when feeling tired or cold. Do not swim at night or on your own. When swimming somewhere unfamiliar, look out for warning notices of tides and strong undercurrents, which indicate those parts of the beach from which it is dangerous to swim. Children must be supervised by an adult who is prepared to go into the water at once if the child is in trouble.

Remember that inflatable mattresses and dinghies are difficult to control. Offshore winds and currents can swiftly carry them out to sea.

Sailing
You must be a confident swimmer and wear a life jacket at all times. Before sailing make sure that the boat is properly equipped and that you (or some other member of the crew) are competent to sail it. It should carry distress flares and a first aid kit. A motorboat should have a fire extinguisher, and a sailing dinghy should be equipped with a set of oars. Before setting out obtain the latest weather forecast. If you are going any distance, let somebody responsible on shore know where you are going and your expected time of arrival, and let that person know when you arrive.

Waterskiing
Safety in waterskiing largely depends on the driver of the boat, who should steer clear of swimmers and other inshore water-users as well as keeping well away from buoys and rocks. Skiers should always wear a life jacket and clothing that is suitable for the weather conditions. Release the rope as soon as you feel yourself falling, curl up into a ball to prevent yourself falling forwards, and once you are in the water collect your skis as soon as possible.

Canoeing
Always wear a life jacket and clothing suitable for the weather conditions. It is important to be properly trained before canoeing so that you know how to react when you capsize. Always go with a companion on canoeing trips and let someone responsible know where you are heading and how long you expect to take; remember to report back to that person when you have arrived. Check the weather forecast before you leave, for sudden rainstorms may transform rivers into dangerous torrents. It is essential that your canoe be properly equipped with toggles, deck lines, adequate buoyancy bags, and a spare paddle secured to the stern deck.

Underwater swimming, scuba diving etc.
It is essential to know how to use your equipment and to know exactly what you are doing in the water. Never go out on your own. Do not dive if you have a cold or respiratory illness. Many clubs insist on a thorough medical examination before allowing someone to join.

Survival techniques

Basic requirements
Survival depends on an awareness of what may go wrong as much as on life-saving equipment. In the following pages, suggestions are offered which will help anyone caught unexpectedly in a dangerous environment. The kit is minimal and consists only of those things that can be kept in a car, in the bottom of a backpack when walking in the wilds, in a locker of a boat, or in a cabinet at a weekend cottage. Although such a kit provides some necessary aids, the real secrets of survival are practicality, carefulness, and avoiding panic.

A basic survival kit should be simple and compact, and if it is homemade, the experience of making it will be useful if an emergency does actually occur. It should provide shelter, warmth, nourishment and a means of identification.
For shelter, a polythene sack, 2m × 1m (6ft × 3ft), is ideal. Alternatively a specially designed body-shaped bag can be bought. This must be windproof and waterproof. Use a piece of brightly coloured material that is easy to see. Parkas, backpacks and weatherproof bags can all be bought in bright colours, such as orange or red. In a flat landscape, tie a piece of bright material to the top of a long stick or pole so that it can be used as a flag.
For warmth, carry matches (but not safety matches) and a piece of sandpaper in a sealed waterproof container. Also carry some material that is easy to light even when moist. A candle helps to conserve the supply of matches. Some types of cigarette lighter are designed for outdoor use; a lighter filled with gasoline rather than with gas is preferable. Make sure it is filled before starting a journey.
For nourishment, carry food to last 24 hours. Include plenty of sugar, chocolate, nuts and raisins, and a few salt tablets.

Even in a cold, wet environment, carry a supply of water. Other highly condensed foods include stock cubes that can be mixed with a small quantity of water, condensed milk, sold in a tube, and extra glucose or dextrose tablets.

For identification, use bright materials, a flashing mirror, a whistle, and smoke from a fire to attract attention.

Additional items that are useful if space permits include a roll of coarse string, a rustproof knife, a flashlight, safety pins, a roll of strong adhesive tape, about 4m (4yds) of strong but fine-gauge wire, a mirror made of steel (not glass), a loud whistle and a reliable compass. If a magnetized piece of metal is used as a compass, remember to mark which end points north. Although these suggestions cover basic requirements, take other items if possible, as mentioned, where appropriate, in the following pages. See also HIKING WITH SAFETY: Checklist – Backpack survival kit.

Survival in cold

The greatest danger to a walker or a climber who is caught in bad weather comes from hypothermia (exposure). This is particularly dangerous because cold and tiredness cause mental confusion, which prevents the victim from noticing the early symptoms of exposure, such as slurred speech and lethargy, that precede unconsciousness, coma and eventually death. It is of vital importance to recognize this lethargy and to oppose it by keeping active and awake. When these symptoms appear, the body needs warmth urgently. The person must drink warm liquids and be moved to safety at once. As a temporary measure, while waiting to be rescued, the body warmth of someone else may also help a person suffering from hypothermia.

Anyone planning to travel in cold conditions must take adequate clothing. In addition to the clothes that are worn, carry an extra sweater, a windproof garment that must be waterproof, a woollen hat, woollen gloves (preferably mittens) and a spare pair of long woollen socks. Wool is the best material, although some synthetic fabrics are also adequate. Cotton, even denim, offers no protection against wind and rain. All items of clothing must be large enough to cover the body. Shirts must be long enough to cover the small of the back and must also have long sleeves. Jackets, trousers and shoes must also be large enough so as not to restrict movement or the circulation of blood. Shoes must be waterproof, with strong, cleated, non-slip soles. Some protection for the eyes, e.g. dark glasses, is necessary in snowy conditions.

Survival in the cold depends first of all on keeping warm. The wind is the greatest threat, so find a place of shelter. Get into the large polythene sack from the emergency kit as soon as convenient. Shelter behind a wall if possible, but avoid ditches or hollows that may fill with water. Use a plastic or nylon sheet to improvise a tent or shelter. If this is brightly coloured it will also help to attract rescuers. Use other emergency equipment to light a fire at night. Keep as dry as possible, since dry clothes minimize heat loss.

If stranded by a snowfall, do not try to walk in the snow,

as the effort will be particularly tiring. Keep warm by moving about in one place, but avoid sweating. If you are covered by snow, whether in a natural shelter or in a car, make sure that you do not suffocate for lack of ventilation or because the roof of the shelter falls in. A stable shelter can be improvised by using slabs of frozen snow to build a thick wall and by roofing this with branches and more snow. When the snowfall ceases, leave a piece of brightly coloured material on the surface to attract rescuers, and do not let this be covered if snow falls again. Build a fire that is sheltered from the wind. Eat small amounts of food regularly.

Surviving heat and drought
Body fluids are lost rapidly in hot conditions. Survival demands that this loss be minimized and, if possible, replaced. Water is much more important for survival in such conditions than food.

Preserve body fluids by keeping as much as possible of the skin covered. Despite the feeling of warmth, much less water is lost as sweat than if the skin is exposed. The head should also be covered. Avoid unnecessary exertion and if possible rest in the shade during the day and travel at night.

If no other water is available a small supply of drinkable water can be obtained by means of a simple solar still. This consists of a hollow in the ground that is completely covered by a stretched plastic sheet. Place a receptacle such as a cup or bowl in the hollow beneath the sheet and put a stone on top of the sheet directly above this bowl. Moisture is evaporated from the ground by the heat of the sun and condenses on the underside of the plastic sheet. The condensation droplets flow down to the point created by the weight of the stone and drip into the bowl directly below. Putting undrinkable fluid (such as seawater, radiator fluid or urine) or even green plants into the hollow increases the moisture of the air beneath the sheet and so increases the quantity of condensation and fresh water that is produced.

Survival in water
If you cannot swim, you should not go near streams, rivers, ponds, lakes or the sea without a life jacket, because someone who cannot swim has little chance of survival in situations that are dangerous even for competent swimmers. The only way a non-swimmer can stay afloat without a life belt or other form of support is to learn to lift the head above water, take a deep breath, close the eyes and float with the face under water until more air is required. Lift the head up, push down with the arms and take another deep breath. Do not try to keep the face above water all the time because this is too tiring.

This technique is also the best way a swimmer can keep afloat. Remember that clothes and shoes become heavy when waterlogged and should be removed. If there is a current, swim with it or across it, but not against it.

If you are in a boat that has capsized, hold on to it or to any part of it that floats, such as the oars. If you become tired, tie yourself to the floating object in case you fall asleep and lose hold. If the boat is floating properly but you are lost, keep the bows or stern pointing into the waves to prevent swamping. Collect rainwater in any available receptacle, including the sails, and use as little fresh water as possible. Never drink seawater. Improvise fishing tackle with string and bent wire.

Surviving in the wild

Some types of vegetation can be eaten but many are harmful if not actually poisonous. Any strange plant that might be edible should be tested by smell, appearance of sap, and initial taste. Plants with an unpleasant smell, a milky sap or a bitter taste should be avoided. If in any doubt at all about the safety of eating a plant, stay hungry and avoid it.

Fish can be caught with a net made from a thin piece of clothing and a forked branch of a tree, and with practice a fishhook and line can be improvised. Dawn and dusk are the best times for fishing, and fish can sometimes be attracted by a light.

Animal snares can be made from thin wire formed into a loop and tied to a tree or bush in a place where the animals are likely to pass. Learn to identify burrows and runs that are in regular use. Most fish and animal flesh can be eaten raw if necessary but meat spoils quickly and should not be kept.

Lightning

During a thunderstorm, the places that are most likely to be struck by lightning are solitary trees and tall objects. A person standing in the open, particularly on a skyline, is vulnerable and someone sheltering beneath an overhanging cliff or in the mouth of a cave is also in danger.

It is safest to shelter inside a building, deep in a cave or in a wood, but not against a tree trunk. If there is no shelter, lie down on flat ground or on the side of a slope.

Surviving a hold-up or hijack

Most important of all, appear calm and do as you are told. Do not answer back to anyone with a weapon, do not appear to disagree or criticize, avoid sudden or suspicious movements and keep your hands visible and your posture relaxed. Avoid eye-contact with the attacker, and do not talk to your companions unless you have been told you may do so. If shooting occurs, lie flat on the floor.

Escape

In general it is safer to remain where you are than to try to escape. This is as true for a hijack or hold-up as it is for a situation in which you are lost and alone. Only if you are in imminent danger or if there is no likelihood of being discovered should you move.

In the wild, it is important to wait in a place that is visible from the air. It is very dangerous to attempt to travel on foot in arctic conditions. In a desert, or even in a hot climate such as jungle, it is better to travel at night and to spend the daylight hours resting. When resting in the shade, leave some visible signal in the open nearby to attract rescuers.

General advice

Always carry a map and compass when travelling away from civilization. Before you set off, make sure that some-one knows the route you intend to follow and the alternative or escape route you will use if something goes wrong. Do not stray from these routes. When travelling in open country, always travel in the same direction. A compass or the stars can be used to help you keep a straight course. Follow water downstream, but don't get too close to the bank. When unsure of your way, mark trees or other objects you pass so that you can retrace your steps if necessary, and remember that it is unwise to travel too far each day, not only because this may make you too tired for the next day but also because you will need time and energy each evening to make a shelter, find food and light a fire.

First aid

You should always carry a basic first aid kit that contains, as a minimum, two triangular bandages, several large Band-Aids, antiseptic cream and several sterile gauze pads. A wide roll of adhesive tape is an alternative, but if this is carried, scissors are also required. A small container of antibiotic powder is useful to prevent wounds becoming septic, especially if you are likely to be away from base for more than 24 hours. A dozen medium-sized safety pins are necessary for securing bandages and for repairing torn clothing.

Signals for help

A fire can be used to produce smoke by day and a source of illumination at night. Be very careful if using this method in woodland. Collect both dry wood and damp leaves so that the former can be added to the fire at night and the latter during the day. On open ground, three fires in a triangle form an international rescue sign.

It is also possible to write on open ground. The letters 'SOS' can be formed with stones or any material that stands out against the ground beneath. In soft ground, the letters can be dug in the form of trenches.

A flag on a long pole is useful in open country or at sea because it is likely to be more visible at a distance than a person waving a flag.

If other people are nearby but appear not to have seen you, their attention can be attracted by whistling or shouting, or by flashing a light. Six even blasts on a whistle over the space of a minute followed by a minute of silence is an international rescue sign. Flashing a light is the best way to attract an aircraft or a ship. In order to direct a beam of reflected sunlight, hold the mirror in front of your face, point your finger at the person you wish to attract and tilt the mirror so that the sunlight hits your extended fingertip.

Domestic accident prevention

More accidents occur in the home than anywhere else, particularly to children and old people. This page lists the main danger areas and suggests how accidents may be prevented. Even when your own home is safe, remember that other houses that your children visit may not be so safe. These same safety principles also apply when on vacation.

Hall passage stairs
1. Well-lit steps to entrances
2. No rug on a polished floor
3. Well-lit stairs
4. Carpet on stairs well-fixed
5. Light switches top and bottom of stairs
6. Gates at top and bottom
7. Sturdy bannister rail
8. No obstacles on the stairs

Living room
9. No trailing flex
10. Fireguard attached to wall
11. Carpets in good repair
12. No mirror over the fire

Kitchen
13. Non-slip floor
14. Cooker with firmly attached pan guards
15. Lockable cabinets for cleaning fluids
16. Cabinets out of children's reach
17. Waste disposal bin of a type that children cannot open
18. Lockable washing machine
19. CO_2 fire extinguisher

Bedroom
20. Heater that cannot burn furniture or curtains
21. Electric blanket in good order and properly earthed
22. Fire escape
23. Never smoke in bed

Nursery (child's room)
24. Cot should be high-sided and stable. No mobiles over the cot. No pillows in the cot
25. Toys should be too large for a child to put in the mouth
26. Safety bars on window

Bathroom
27. Handrails by bath and toilet
28. All electric fittings should have cord switches and be placed high up, away from the bath
29. Medicine cabinet lockable and out of a child's reach
30. Non-slip mats on the floor and in the bath

In all parts of the house, fit electric sockets with childproof safety covers. Keep electric fittings in good repair and replace wires that are worn. All appliances should be earthed and have correct fuses.

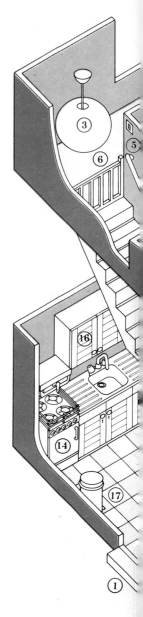

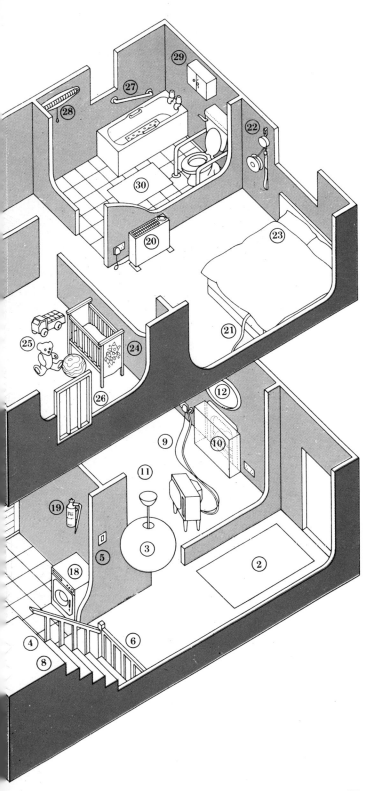

Good health and fitness

Good health depends on many factors. Lifestyle, eating habits, use of drugs and ways of relaxation may all affect general health. In the following pages, advice is offered about common hazards to health that can be avoided, and about ways in which health of mind and body can best be maintained.

The causes of ill health

People who work hard and competitively for personal fulfilment or financial gain lead stressful lives. In certain cases their working day may be so full of tension that they are unable to relax sufficiently at home in the evenings and at night. Difficult travelling conditions on the way to work, pressure in work itself and frustration if work has been unsatisfactorily done can contribute to illnesses such as stomach ulcer, heart attack or nervous disorder.

Stress is harmful to the body because it disrupts the normal patterns of physiological and biochemical activity. Certain endocrine and lymphatic glands may overwork and others may work too little in a person who is under stress. The digestive system, particularly the stomach, reacts poorly to variations in metabolic requirements and the heart and circulation are damaged by the excessive demands placed on them. A person living under stress is more likely to make use of artificial stimulants and sedatives than someone living a quieter life. Such a person is likely to be more interested in meals that can be prepared quickly than in foods that constitute a more correctly balanced diet. Someone whose lifestyle allows little time for relaxation is also likely to have too little time to take adequate exercise.

Clarifying one's priorities, even if this means taking a less aggressive or competitive stance at work, is likely to benefit general health. If the job is too important, health can be improved by identifying the potential dangers and compensating for them by paying special attention to other health-improving factors such as taking regular exercise, eating a balanced diet, and avoiding alcohol, tobacco and other drugs.

Diet

For good health it is important to have the correct body weight for your age, sex and build. Being overweight is a proven hazard. In addition to putting extra strain on the joints, heart and circulation, excess fat probably indicates that too much rich food (which is high in cholesterol) is being eaten. A high level of cholesterol in the blood may cause deterioration of the arteries and so increase the risk of thrombosis.

A healthy diet must contain a variety of types of food. Carbohydrates, proteins, fats, vitamins and minerals are required in varying proportions. Vitamins and minerals are essential but are only required in minute quantities. Fats give the most energy but they may also cause ill health through blood vessel disease. Proteins are necessary for growth. The basic protein elements (amino acids) may be obtained from many foods including cereals, vegetables and nuts; a varied diet ensures that all the necessary amino acids are present. Carbohydrates occur in various forms and are the basis of most people's diet. They are primarily a source of energy, but some types of carbohydrate also form the roughage (fibre bulk) that is required if the bowel muscles are to function properly.

Eating a balanced diet is essential to any programme for maintaining good health. Most people eat too much and many eat the wrong things. It is probable that the desire to overeat disappears if the diet is restricted to those foods that are best suited to the body's requirements. Sugar (a carbohydrate) and animal fats should be avoided as much as possible. Unsweetened fruit juices, water and bulky fibre foods are generally beneficial. Starch (also a carbohydrate), which is the chief constituent of potatoes and bread, is a necessary part of any diet and a moderate intake of starchy carbohydrate will not lead to obesity. Many of the nutritional components of potatoes and other vegetables are found in their skins. The whole grain of wheat that is used in wholewheat bread is more nutritious than the refined flour used to make white bread, and this should be remembered if bread and potatoes make up a large part of the diet.

The small quantities of essential vitamins and minerals that the body requires are provided by most diets that contain a variety of foods such as vegetables, milk, eggs, fruit and meat. If vegetables are boiled some vitamins are destroyed by heat or lost because they are water-soluble. In affluent countries many foods contain additional vitamins and for this reason ill health due to vitamin deficiency is rare. A deficiency of iron does sometimes occur in women because of heavy menstruation. If this occurs, listlessness and other symptoms of iron-deficiency anemia may appear. It has been suggested that large quantities of some vitamins, particularly vitamin C, may help to prevent and may indeed speed recovery from illness, but at present scientific opinion is divided on this question.

The types of dietary fats that are potentially harmful include the saturated fats and cholesterol. The term 'saturated' refers to the chemical structure of the fat molecules. The degrees of saturation are relative. Most animal fats are saturated and typically appear solid when cold. Unsaturated fats are obtained primarily from plants and fish and are usually liquid. Cholesterol is produced by the human body and is necessary for the formation of new tissues, but an excess of cholesterol in the blood leads to its being deposited in the walls of arteries and damaging these vessels.

Obesity is a serious hazard to health. In an older person it can be as dangerous as regular smoking. The appearance of loose fatty flesh around the face, upper arms, chest, waist or thighs is the most obvious indication of obesity. A table of ideal weights may also prove useful provided that natural variations such as sex, build and age are taken into account. The table below estimates the ideal naked weight of a 30-year-old person of average build. A person of heavy or light build should add or subtract 3kg (7lbs) from the weight given and anyone between the ages of 20 and 45 should add or subtract 0.5kg (1lb) for each year that they are older or younger than 30. The table covers a middle range of heights and anyone not covered by this range should add or subtract 2kg (4lbs) for each inch of difference.

Height	cm	160	163	165	168	170	173	175	178	180	183
	feet	5'3"	5'4"	5'5"	5'6"	5'7"	5'8"	5'9"	5'10"	5'11"	6'0"
Male	kg	61.2	63.0	64.9	66.7	68.5	70.3	72.1	73.9	75.7	77.6
Weight	lbs	135	139	143	147	151	155	159	163	167	171
Female	kg	57.1	59.0	60.9	62.6	64.4	66.2	68.0	69.8	71.7	73.5
Weight	lbs	126	130	134	138	142	146	150	154	158	162

No table of this kind can do more than offer a rough guide to the correct weight of a person who has a particular height and build, but in general it may be assumed that anyone who differs from the weight calculated from this table by more than 10–15% is probably over- or underweight. Such a person should consult a doctor for further advice.

If you need to lose weight, ask your doctor for advice about a suitable diet that takes into account any medical problems you may have and that supplements any nutrients that may be lacking.

In nearly all cases the body puts on fat because the amount of food eaten is greater than the amount of energy being used up. The basis of any successful slimming programme is the correct balance between the intake and the output of energy. The easiest way an overweight person can improve this balance is to eat less and to take more exercise. It is also important to be selective in the choice of food because the energy obtained from some foods (such as fats) is so much greater than from others (such as proteins) that fewer of the high-energy foods are required.

Exercise
Regular exercise is essential for good health and is particularly important for preventing heart and lung disorders. It increases physical strength, suppleness and stamina, and often encourages mental alertness as well as physical agility. Exercise also improves the complexion and gives confidence in posture and movement.

A systematic programme of physical exercise should not be too ambitious initially. A ten-minute jog each day, just fast enough to produce breathlessness and to increase the pulse rate without strain, brings about a dramatic improvement in the health of most people, especially those who have sedentary jobs. Jogging can easily be combined with other daily obligations such as walking the dog or returning home after taking the children to nursery school. As an alternative to jogging, a game such as tennis or badminton, or swimming at least twice a week, also helps to maintain physical fitness in ways that are pleasant and do not require a large amount of self-discipline.

Specific exercises are particularly valuable for improving the strength and shape of different parts of the body. Exercising the abdominal muscles helps to reduce stomach fat. Running or step-up exercises strengthen the legs. Exercising the waist muscles gives the waist a better shape. These exercises can be developed from the range of warm-up exercises that are used by athletes to prepare their muscles for strenuous activity.

People who take little exercise may find that their muscles and joints lose suppleness and strength. For such people exercising neck, shoulder, arm, chest, back, waist, hip, leg and ankle muscles for a few minutes each day will greatly improve the feeling of general physical health.

Relaxation
In addition to taking regular exercise many people also need to learn how to relax. One of the best ways of relaxing is to develop an interest or hobby outside the contexts of work and family. Such interests are relaxing because they distract from the pressures of life without necessarily creating stressful demands themselves.

There is more to relaxing than simply getting enough sleep and physical rest, and in general it is probably true to say that the mental aspects of relaxation are even more important than the physical. Hobbies and vacations alone are not enough to solve the problem for many people, especially if there are persistent causes of anxiety. For this and other reasons the use of mental or spiritual exercises such as meditation to aid relaxation is becoming increasingly common. There are many schools of meditation advocating different techniques in order to achieve the desired states of relaxation or spiritual peace. Another Eastern discipline that is popular in the West is yoga, which is often found to be particularly valuable because of the ways in which it combines exercises to relieve physical tension with techniques that help to relieve mental stress.

The text above has suggested how good health can be encouraged and maintained. More detailed advice on these topics can be obtained from a doctor, and specialists in the appropriate field can also be consulted.

Care of the sick at home

Caring for someone recovering from an illness, an old person or a member of the family who may be ill for some time can be made more pleasant for the sick (as well as for the healthy) if it is done at home. Whether the sickroom is the patient's own bedroom or another more convenient room in the house, there are certain basic requirements, and there are also many helpful techniques that can contribute to the comfort of the patient, to the convenience of the nurse and to the general wellbeing of the whole household.

Basic requirements

The basic requirements of a sickroom are a comfortable bed with a firm mattress and additional pillows, in a well-ventilated room at a comfortable temperature. A non-slip floor will also help. Remove any rugs from beside the bed. Put a chair near the bed as an aid to getting out of bed and for the patient to sit on if necessary.

The bedside table should have a jug of water and a glass, a hand-bell or electric bell for the patient to call for help if necessary, and a reading light that can be dimmed at night. There should be a toilet nearby and there should also be a vomit bowl if necessary.

Taking a temperature: mouth

Shake the thermometer so that the reading is below minimum on the scale and place the thermometer under the patient's tongue. Ask the patient to close the lips around the thermometer and leave it there for at least two minutes. Remove the thermometer, read the mercury level and write down the reading. Shake the thermometer so that the mercury level falls below minimum again. Clean the bulb with antiseptic before putting it away in its case.

Taking a temperature: rectum

This method is generally used for babies. Grease the end of the thermometer with petroleum jelly. Lay the baby on its back, hold its feet in the air, and insert the bulb of the thermometer just inside the rectum. Leave it in place for at least two minutes. Remove the thermometer, read the temperature and write down the reading. The rectal temperature is usually about 0.5°C (1°F) higher than the temperature taken in the mouth.

Diet and fluids

A feverish patient requires more fluid than usual and must be encouraged to drink at least 2 litres (4 pints) of liquid a day. Solid food can be a problem because most bed-ridden patients have a poor appetite. Food should be appetizing and nutritious and small portions should be given.

Vomiting

To help someone who is vomiting, support the forehead with one hand and hold a bowl in the other. When vomiting has ceased, sponge the patient's face and forehead with cool water and rinse the patient's mouth.

Drugs

Keep drugs away from the patient's reach to prevent accidental overdosage. Give only as directed by the doctor.

Giving a bed bath

The key principle is to wash one part of the patient at a time, keeping the rest of the body covered with a thick towel or a blanket to prevent the patient getting cold. The sequence should be:

1. Put a large towel under the patient, then cover the patient and wash and dry the face and neck. **2.** Wash and dry each arm and the adjacent side of the chest, completing one side before starting the other. **3.** Cover the chest and arms before washing and drying the abdomen and groin. **4.** Wash each leg, keeping the rest of the body covered. **5.** Roll the patient onto the side and wash the back. Throughout washing it is important to dry the skin thoroughly and to powder creases, particularly under the breasts, in the groin and between the buttocks.

Care of the mouth
The patient should rinse the mouth with a mouth wash after meals and brush the teeth at least twice a day. False teeth must be cleaned regularly. Dry lips should be moistened with a lip salve.

Care of hair and nails
Hair should be brushed and combed at least twice a day. Nails must be kept clean and cut regularly.

Humidity
The sickroom should not be too dry, because dry air may aggravate coughing or cause discomfort to breathing. Humidity may be increased by leaving large bowls of water in the room or by boiling a kettle in the room (away from the bed).

Blanket supports

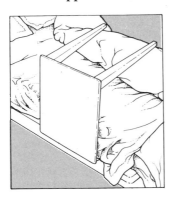 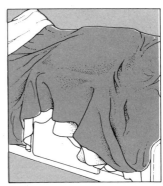

Blanket supports are used to take the weight of the bed-clothes off the patient's legs. A temporary support can be made by using a stool on its side and inserting its lower legs under the mattress.

Nose drops
Make sure the patient is sitting or lying comfortably with the head tilted back. Draw up liquid in a dropper and insert the dropper into a nostril. Release the number of drops prescribed and repeat in the other nostril. Ask the patient to sniff to inhale the drops.

Eye drops

Make sure the patient is sitting or lying comfortably with the head tilted back. Stand behind and with one hand pull the lower eyelid gently downwards. Rest the other hand, holding the dropper, on the patient's forehead. Insert the drops exactly as prescribed between the eye and the lowered lid. Repeat into the other eye. Ask the patient to blink several times.

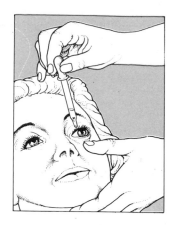

Problems of old age

Old age is not a sudden occurrence like puberty. It is a gradual change in the normal working of the body, a continuation of the processes that have been occurring throughout life. This change may be more rapid in some people than in others. In a healthy person, aging seems to depend largely on genetic factors: for example, members of some families live longer than those of others.

In the text below, words in italics refer to subjects to be found in the A–Z OF DISEASES, SYMPTOMS AND TREATMENTS. Alternatively, look for the subjects in the INDEX.

The normal changes of aging. Old age is accompanied by various changes in the body which produce slower physical reactions. There is a gradual deterioration of vision, partly due to changes in the eye lens such as *cataracts* and *farsightedness*, and partly due to the failure of the light-sensitive cells in the retina. *Deafness* is also a common occurrence due to a similar degeneration of the nerve cells.

Healthy senior citizens generally lead active physical lives but may find difficulty in understanding or accepting new ideas. They require almost as much food as a younger adult and need just as much sleep, although the pattern may be changed by sleeping more during the day and less at night. They usually have less stamina: fatigue occurs more quickly unless a regular pattern of activity is maintained.

Disease in old age. Elderly people who are healthy have good resistance to many of the everyday infectious illnesses, such as the common *cold* or *influenza*, because they have acquired immunity from many previous infections. If, however, they do become ill it is likely to be more serious and to last longer than if they were younger. Immediate treatment of a respiratory illness may prevent it developing into *bronchitis* or *pneumonia*.

Many physical disorders occur in old age because of deterioration of a particular organ or part of the body. This can be seen in blood vessels, due to *arteriosclerosis*, which may lead to a *stroke* or *heart attack*. These blood vessel disorders are made worse by high *blood pressure*. People suffering from *obesity* are more likely to develop *diabetes* or hyperthyroidism (see *Thyroid problems*), both glandular disorders that are more likely in old age; the latter increases the risk of hypothermia in cold weather. *Arthritis* occurs to some degree in all elderly people, and urinary disorders, due to *prostate problems* in men or, in women, *prolapse of the womb,* may cause *incontinence.*

Unfortunately, once things start to go wrong with an elderly person the ability to cope rapidly disappears. Illness may cause confusion and this, combined with forgetfulness, leads to a poor diet, inactivity and loneliness. *Constipation* is a common problem.

As the general health of an elderly person deteriorates so the social problem increases. Many families may find themselves unable to cope with the burden. It is important to consult your doctor early and to take full advantage of the many facilities that the social services can provide. Sometimes a short period in a hospital not only helps the patient but also relieves the family, allowing them perhaps to take a vacation and return ready to cope once again.

Care of an elderly patient. The elderly must be encouraged to do things for themselves. Regular bathing or bed bathing is important, with careful drying and powdering of the skin folds. Hair should be brushed daily and washed weekly. Foot care is important, and *corns* and *bunions* require podiatry. The mouth, particularly the teeth and gums, needs rinsing, and dental treatment and properly fitting dentures may be a necessary part of oral hygiene. Encourage regular bowel movements, but use only the mildest laxatives or glycerine suppositories when necessary. Sedative drugs to aid sleep may cause confusion: use only when a doctor feels they are really necessary. Regular exercise maintains muscle strength and joint movements.

Checklist – Household aids for the elderly

City, state and federal social agencies are often able to provide needed financial support as well as professional aid and counselling services to help the elderly in health maintenance.

In the bathroom: a handrail by the bath; a rail over the taps; a non-slip mat in the bath; a special seat in the bath; a handrail by the toilet; and a long-handled toothbrush.

In the bedroom: a high bed, because it is easier to get out of than a low one; a firm mattress or a board under the mattress; a commode by the bedside; a blanket support to go over the feet; and a bell by the bedside.

For clothing: self-adhesive fasteners, instead of buttons or hooks; a front-opening bra; a long-handled shoehorn; special stocking aids to help pull stockings on; slip-on shoes; non-slip soles on shoes; and clip-on ties and braces.

In the kitchen: a wall can-opener; trays with non-slip surfaces and a spiked board for cutting vegetables.

For eating: unspillable cups; plate grips on the table and thickened handles on utensils (made by taping foam rubber or attaching plastic around them).

For home lighting: wall sockets placed 1.25m (4ft) above the floor; switches with lengthened handles; rubber balls attached to the ends of pull switches; and good reading lights.

For door handles: levers are easier to turn than knobs.

MEDICAL ENCYCLOPEDIA

Introduction

This section of the book is a small encyclopedia filled with useful information: how MEDICAL WORDS are built from their Greek and Latin roots, to help you understand medical terms; HOW THE BODY WORKS, explaining with clear illustrations and simple text how human anatomy and physiology work; and simple diagrammatic CHARTS OF WHAT TO DO, to help you decide what action to take if you have a common complaint, such as a headache or chest pain.

The major part of this section is the A–Z OF DISEASES, SYMPTOMS AND TREATMENTS, describing many conditions about which you or your family may want to know. The section ends with information about MEDICINAL DRUGS.

Medical words

At first glance, the jargon of a science may seem to be the hardest part of the subject to understand. In medicine, however, most terms are constructed from elements that have simple meanings, usually derived from words in Greek or Latin. The following list gives the basic meaning of some of these elements and examples of their use.

Element	Meaning	Example
a, an	without	*an*uria: without passing urine
ab, apo	away from	*ab*normal: other than normal
ad	towards	*ad*renal: towards the kidney
aden-i-o	gland	*aden*iform: gland-shaped
alg-e-ia-y	pain	an*alge*sia: without pain
andro	male	*andro*cyte: male (sex) cell
angi-o	vessel	*angio*gram: X-ray of a blood vessel
ant-i	against	*anti*septic: against bacterial decay
ante	before	*ante*natal: before birth
arteri-o	artery	*arterio*sclerosis: hardening of an artery
arthr-o	joint	*arthr*itis: joint inflammation
auto	self	*auto*hypnosis: self-induced hypnosis
bili	bile	*bili*ary: of the bile
blephar-o	eyelid	*blephar*itis: eyelid inflammation
brachi-o	arm	*brachi*al: of the arm
brady	slow	*brady*cardia: slow heartbeat
bronch-i-o	bronchus	*broncho*spasm: spasm of bronchial tubes in the lungs
carcin-o	cancer	*carcino*genic: cancer-producing
cardi-o	heart	*cardio*logy: study of the heart

cata,cath	down	*cata*rrh: flowing down of mucus
cel-e-i-o	abdomen	*cel*iac: abdominal
cephal-o	head	*cephalo*metry: head measurement
cerebr-o	brain	*cerebr*al: of the brain
cervic-o	neck	*cervix*: the neck of the womb
chol-e-ia-o	bile; gall	*chole*cystitis: gall bladder inflammation
chondr-ia-o	cartilage	*chondro*cyte: cartilage cell
col-o-ono	colon	*col*ectomy: excision of the colon
cortic-o	outer layer	adreno*cortic*al: of the adrenal cortex
cost-o	rib	inter*cost*al: between the ribs
cox-o	hip	*cox*algia: pain in the hip
crani-o	skull	*cranio*pathy: disease of the skull
cry-mo-o	cold	*cryo*genic: temperature-lowering
crypt-o	hidden	*crypto*genic: of hidden origin
cut-a-i-icul	skin	*cut*aneous: of the skin
cyst-o	bladder	*cysto*gram: X-ray of the bladder
cyt-e-o	cell	*cyto*toxic: toxic to cells
dent-i-o	tooth	*dent*ition: arrangement of teeth
derm-ato-is-o	skin	*derm*atitis: inflammation of the skin
dipl-o	double	*diplo*pia: double vision
dips-o	thirst	*dipso*maniac: alcoholic
dors-a-i-o	back	*dorsi*flexion: bending backwards
dys	abnormal	*dys*phagia: difficulty in swallowing
ec-to-tasia	outer	*ecto*derm: outer layer of skin
en-do-to	in; inside	*endo*crinal: secreting internally
enter-o	intestine	*enter*itis: intestinal inflammation
ep-i	outside	*epi*dermis: outermost layer of skin
erythr-o	red	*erythro*cyte: red (blood) cell
esthe	sensation	an*esthe*sia: without feeling
ex	out	*ex*crete: evacuate
extra	outside	*extra*vascular: outside a vessel
galact-o	milk	*galact*orrhea: excessive flow of milk
gastr-o	stomach	*gastr*itis: inflammation of the stomach
ger-ia-o	old age	*geria*tric: of old age
gloss-o	tongue	*gloss*al: of the tongue
glyc-o	sugar	*glyc*emia: sugar in the blood
gyn-e-eco	female	*gyneco*logy: study of female disorders

hem-a-at-o	blood	*hemat*uria: blood in the urine
hemi	half	*hemi*plegia: paralysis of half the body
hepat-o	liver	*hepat*itis: inflammation of the liver
heter-o	different	*hetero*geneous: of different kind
homo-eo-o	same	*homo*genous: of the same origin
hyper	over	*hyper*active: overactive
hypn-o	sleep	*hypn*otic: inducing sleep
hypo	under	*hypo*thermia: lack of heat
hyster-o	womb	*hyster*ectomy: removal of the womb
iatr-o-y	medicine	*iatro*genic: caused by medicine
ile-o	of the ileum	*ile*itis: inflammation of the ileum (part of the intestine)
ili-o	of the ilium	*ili*ac: of the ilium (bone in the pelvic girdle)
infra	below	*infra*-axillary: below the armpit
intr-à-o	within	*intra*gastric: within the stomach
iso	equal	*iso*morphous: having the same form
itis	inflammation	ir*itis*: inflammation of the iris
kin-e-eto	movement	*kineto*genic: causing movement
lab-i-io-r	lip	*labi*al: of the lips
lact-i-o	milk	*lact*ation: the secretion of milk
lapse	fall	pro*lapse*: falling forward
leuco (leuko)	white	*leuko*cyte: white blood cell
lingu-a	tongue	sub*lingual*: under the tongue
lip-id-o	fat; fatty	*lip*emia: fat in the blood
lith-ia-o	stone	nephro*lith*: kidney stone
ly-o-sis-so	dissolving	lipo*lysis*: dissolution of fat
lymph-o	lymph	*lymph*atic: of lymph or lymph vessels
malacia-o	softness	osteo*malacia*: softening of the bones
mamm-a-o	breast	*mamma*ry: of the breast
mast-o	breast	*mast*itis: inflammation of the breast
mega-lo-ly	great	*megalo*cyte: enlarged red blood cell
men-o-s	monthly	dys*meno*rrhea: painful menstruation
metr-ia-o	womb	*metr*itis: inflammation of the womb
my-o	muscle	*myo*cardial: muscular cardiac tissue
myel-o	marrow	*myelo*ma: tumour of bone marrow
narco-tico	numbness	*narco*tic: producing stupor

nas-a-o	nose	*naso*pharynx: nasal part of the pharynx
necro	death	*necro*phobia: fear of death
neo	new	*neo*natal: newly born
nephr-o	kidney	*nephr*itis: inflammation of the kidney
ocul-o	eye	*ocul*ist: eye specialist
onych-ia-o	nail	*onycho*lysis: destruction of nail
oo, ovi, ovo	egg; ovum	*oo*cyte: egg cell
ophthalm-o	eye	*ophthalm*itis: inflammation of the eye
op-tic-to	eye	*optic*ian: eye specialist
orth-o	straight	*orth*optics: straightening vision
os-se-teo	bone	*osteo*metry: measurement of bones
ot-i-ico-o	ear	*ot*itis: inflammation of the ear
par-esis	weakness	myo*paresis*: muscle weakness
par-ous-a	bearing	multi*parous*: having many offspring
path-e-o-y	disease	*patho*logy: study of disease
pector-i	chest	*pectoral*is major: a muscle of the chest
ped-ia-o	child	*pedia*trician: children's doctor
penia	lack	leuco*penia*: lack of white blood cells
pep-sia-t	digestion	*pep*tic ulcer: stomach ulcer
peri	round	*peri*cellular: surrounding a cell
phall-o	penis	*phall*ic: shaped like a penis
pharmac-o	drugs	*pharmaco*logy: study of drugs
pharyng	pharynx	*pharyng*itis: pharyngeal inflammation
phleb	vein	*phleb*itis: inflammation of a vein
phyla-c-ctic	protection	pro*phylactic*: preventive treatment
pleur-o	rib; side	*pleuro*dynia: pain between the ribs
poly	many	*poly*cellular: with many cells
pseud-o	false	*pseudo*pregnancy: false pregnancy
psych-o	mind	*psycho*logy: study of the mind
pulm-o-on	lung	*pulmon*ary: of the lungs
py-o	pus	*pyo*genic: forming pus
ren-i-o	of the kidney	*ren*al calculus: kidney stone
rhin-o	nose	*rhin*itis: inflammation of the nose
rrhag-e-ia	outflow	hemo*rrhage*: outflow of blood
rrhea	outflow	dia*rrhea*: outflow of feces
rube	red	*rube*facient: making red
sarc-o	flesh	*sarc*oma: fleshy tumour

scler-a-o	hardening	*scler*oderma: hardening of the skin
seb-a-i-o	fatty secretion	*sebo*rrhea: excessive secretion of fatty substances
sect, section	cutting	hemi*section*: cutting into two parts
sep-sis-tic	decay	*septic*emia: infection in the blood
sero	of serum	*sero*enzyme: enzyme in the blood serum
som-a-t-to	body	*soma*tic: pertaining to the body
splen-o	spleen	*splen*ectomy: excision of the spleen
spondyl-o	vertebra	*spondyl*algia: pain in a vertebra
stea-to	fat	*steato*rrhea: fat in the feces
steno	contracted	*steno*sis: narrowing
steth-o	chest	*stetho*scope: instrument for examining the chest
sthen-ia-ic	strength	a*sthenia*: loss of strength
stom-a-ato-y	mouth	*stoma*titis: mouth inflammation
syl, sym, syn	with	*syn*ergy: working together
tach-o-eo-y	fast	*tachy*cardia: fast heartbeat
tax-ia-y	co-ordination	a*taxia*: lack of muscular co-ordination
tele	end; far off	*tele*neuron: nerve ending
therap	treatment	*therap*eutics: the science of healing
thorac-ic-o	of the chest	*thoraco*tomy: cutting into the chest
thromb-o-us	blood clot	*thrombo*lytic: dissolving a blood clot
tomy	cutting	hysterec*tomy*: removal of the womb
ton-ia-ic	tension	myo*tonia*: persistent muscle tension
tox-ic-ico	poison	*tox*emia: blood-poisoning
trache-a-o	windpipe	*tracheo*tomy: windpipe surgery
troph-o-y	nutrition	a*trophy*: lack of growth
tympan-o	(ear) drum	*tympan*itis: eardrum inflammation
ur-ino-o	urine	poly*uria*: frequent urination
uter-o	uterus	*uter*itis: uterine inflammation
vagin	vagina	*vagin*itis: vaginal inflammation
vas-i-o	vessel; sperm duct	*vaso*constriction: narrowing of a blood-vessel
vesic-a-o-u	bladder	*vesic*ula: small bladder-like structure
vir-o	virus	*viro*logy: study of viruses
xer-o	dry	*xero*stomia: dryness of the mouth

How the body works – Anatomy and Physiology

Introduction

An understanding of medical disorders and problems, with their symptoms and the ways they are treated, is based on a knowledge of the human body. The systems and various parts of the body are described on the following pages. A complete figure is outlined in each case to show how the system relates to the body as a whole, and the part of the body being described is illustrated separately to show its chief anatomical features.

Muscles, bones and joints are the mechanical structures that give the body its shape and enable it to move. Muscles attach to bones through ligaments and tendons. The forces exerted on bones by the action of muscles cause the bones to move against one another. Joints are the junctions between bones. The joints must be flexible and must have smooth surfaces to prevent friction, yet must be strong enough to prevent the bones from moving the wrong way. See pp.82–83.

The nervous system and the senses control the mechanical functions of the body. The brain collects, co-ordinates, stores and recalls information brought to it by the sensory nerves from receptors such as the eyes, ears, nose and tongue. See pp.84–85.

The heart, circulation and respiration work together to provide the body with oxygenated blood and to remove waste products such as carbon dioxide from the tissues. Blood is oxygenated in the lungs and is pumped round the body by the heart. The tissues absorb the oxygen and other nourishment (from digestion) that they need from the blood. See pp.86–87.

The digestive system breaks down and absorbs as much as possible of everything that is swallowed. The waste is excreted as feces. Cells lining the digestive tract convert substances into a form that can be transported by the blood to the liver and to other tissues where further metabolism takes place. See p.88.

The urinary system includes the two kidneys that filter the blood, remove unwanted waste products of metabolism and regulate the balance of salts and water in the body. Waste products are stored temporarily in the bladder and excreted as urine. See p.89.

The reproductive and endocrine systems are concerned respectively with reproduction and with the production of chemical messengers (hormones). The reproductive systems consist of the internal and external genitalia that produce sperm in the male and eggs (ova) in the female, and provide the conditions in which these can combine and develop. The endocrine glands produce the hormones that control metabolism and regulate the balance of fluids and salts in the blood. Hormones also control development and sexual activity. See p.90.

Muscles, bones and joints

The diagrams on this spread illustrate the principal muscles and bones of the body and the structure of a joint, a bone and a muscle.

The knee joint, from behind, illustrates the relationship between bone and cartilage, and shows how ligaments attach to bones and bind the bones together.

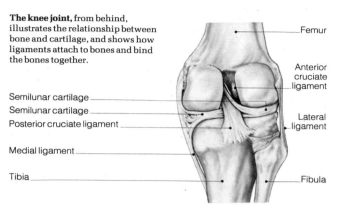

Femur

Anterior cruciate ligament

Semilunar cartilage

Semilunar cartilage

Posterior cruciate ligament

Lateral ligament

Medial ligament

Tibia

Fibula

Muscles and bones of the body

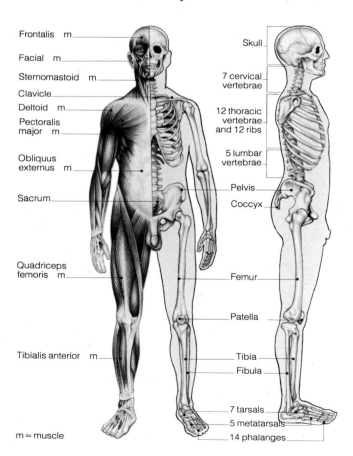

Frontalis m

Facial m

Sternomastoid m

Clavicle

Deltoid m

Pectoralis major m

Obliquus externus m

Sacrum

Quadriceps femoris m

Tibialis anterior m

m = muscle

Skull

7 cervical vertebrae

12 thoracic vertebrae and 12 ribs

5 lumbar vertebrae

Pelvis

Coccyx

Femur

Patella

Tibia

Fibula

7 tarsals

5 metatarsals

14 phalanges

Long bones, such as the femur, are tubes with sponge-like centres filled with marrow at the ends. Blood is formed by marrow, mainly in the flat bones.

Skeletal muscle is under voluntary control. It consists of elongated cells that contract and relax rapidly, when stimulated by motor nerves.

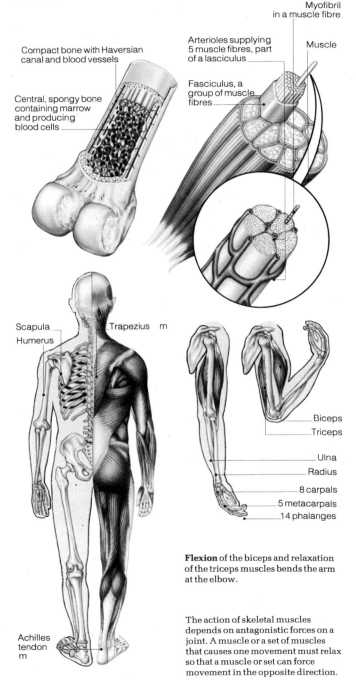

Myofibril in a muscle fibre

Muscle

Compact bone with Haversian canal and blood vessels

Arterioles supplying 5 muscle fibres, part of a lasciculus

Central, spongy bone containing marrow and producing blood cells

Fasciculus, a group of muscle fibres

Scapula
Humerus
Trapezius m

Biceps
Triceps

Ulna
Radius
8 carpals
5 metacarpals
14 phalanges

Achilles tendon m

Flexion of the biceps and relaxation of the triceps muscles bends the arm at the elbow.

The action of skeletal muscles depends on antagonistic forces on a joint. A muscle or a set of muscles that causes one movement must relax so that a muscle or set can force movement in the opposite direction.

Nervous system

The nervous system is regulated by the brain, which receives and sends out messages through the peripheral nerves by way of nerve fibres in the spinal cord.

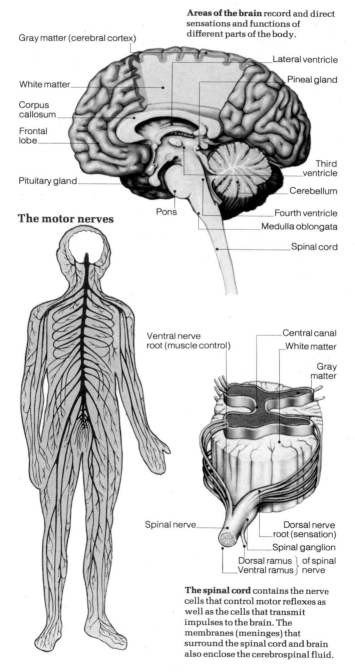

Areas of the brain record and direct sensations and functions of different parts of the body.

Gray matter (cerebral cortex)

Lateral ventricle

Pineal gland

White matter

Corpus callosum

Frontal lobe

Third ventricle

Pituitary gland

Cerebellum

Pons

Fourth ventricle

Medulla oblongata

Spinal cord

The motor nerves

Ventral nerve root (muscle control)

Central canal

White matter

Gray matter

Spinal nerve

Dorsal nerve root (sensation)

Spinal ganglion

Dorsal ramus ⎱ of spinal
Ventral ramus ⎰ nerve

The spinal cord contains the nerve cells that control motor reflexes as well as the cells that transmit impulses to the brain. The membranes (meninges) that surround the spinal cord and brain also enclose the cerebrospinal fluid.

The senses

Sight, hearing, balance, smell and taste senses are each located in specific organs. Senses of touch, temperature and muscular position are in the skin and muscles.

Structure of the eye

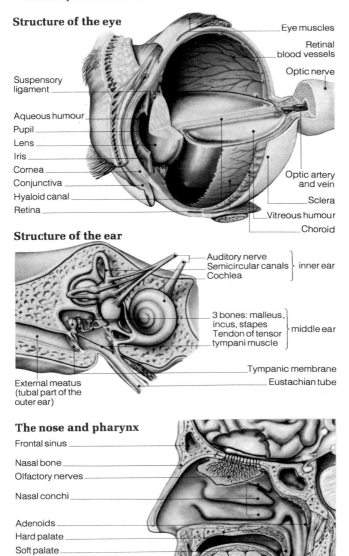

Eye muscles

Retinal blood vessels

Optic nerve

Suspensory ligament

Aqueous humour

Pupil

Lens

Iris

Cornea

Conjunctiva

Hyaloid canal

Retina

Optic artery and vein

Sclera

Vitreous humour

Choroid

Structure of the ear

Auditory nerve
Semicircular canals } inner ear
Cochlea

3 bones: malleus, incus, stapes
Tendon of tensor tympani muscle } middle ear

Tympanic membrane

Eustachian tube

External meatus (tubal part of the outer ear)

The nose and pharynx

Frontal sinus

Nasal bone

Olfactory nerves

Nasal conchi

Adenoids

Hard palate

Soft palate

Tonsil

Tongue

Lingual nerve

Epiglottis

Esophagus

Trachea

Tastes (of sweet, sour and salt) are detected by areas of the tongue.

85

Heart and circulation

The circulating blood supplies the tissues of the body with nutrition (oxygen and food) and removes waste products such as carbon dioxide and urea.

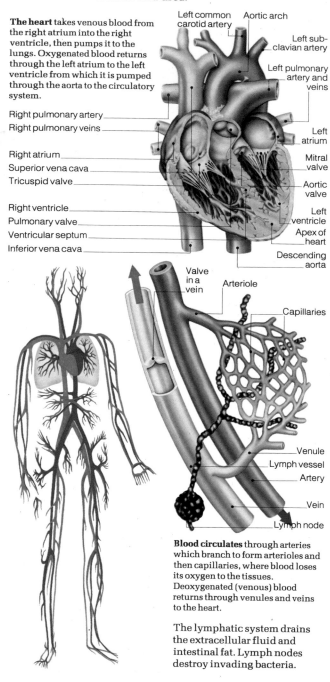

The heart takes venous blood from the right atrium into the right ventricle, then pumps it to the lungs. Oxygenated blood returns through the left atrium to the left ventricle from which it is pumped through the aorta to the circulatory system.

Left common carotid artery
Aortic arch
Left sub-clavian artery
Left pulmonary artery and veins
Right pulmonary artery
Right pulmonary veins
Left atrium
Right atrium
Superior vena cava
Tricuspid valve
Mitral valve
Aortic valve
Right ventricle
Pulmonary valve
Ventricular septum
Inferior vena cava
Left ventricle
Apex of heart
Descending aorta

Valve in a vein
Arteriole
Capillaries
Venule
Lymph vessel
Artery
Vein
Lymph node

Blood circulates through arteries which branch to form arterioles and then capillaries, where blood loses its oxygen to the tissues. Deoxygenated (venous) blood returns through venules and veins to the heart.

The lymphatic system drains the extracellular fluid and intestinal fat. Lymph nodes destroy invading bacteria.

Respiration

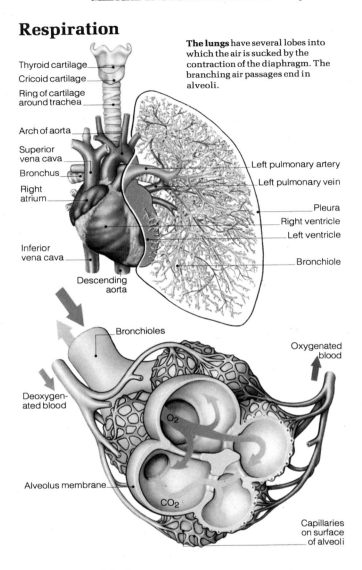

Thyroid cartilage
Cricoid cartilage
Ring of cartilage around trachea
Arch of aorta
Superior vena cava
Bronchus
Right atrium
Inferior vena cava
Descending aorta

The lungs have several lobes into which the air is sucked by the contraction of the diaphragm. The branching air passages end in alveoli.

Left pulmonary artery
Left pulmonary vein
Pleura
Right ventricle
Left ventricle
Bronchiole

Bronchioles
Oxygenated blood
Deoxygenated blood
O_2
Alveolus membrane
CO_2
Capillaries on surface of alveoli

An alveolus of the lungs

Blood-gas exchange occurs in the alveoli of the lungs. Capillaries that surround an alveolus carry blood containing carbon dioxide. Oxygen inside the alveolus passes through the surface membrane and combines with hemoglobin in the red blood cells. Carbon dioxide is released in exchange. Freshly oxygenated blood returns to the heart, and the air that is expired from the lungs carries the waste carbon dioxide with it. Cells lining the bronchioles and bronchi have hairs (cilia) that remove dust and mucus from the lungs.

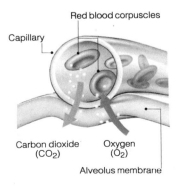

Red blood corpuscles
Capillary
Carbon dioxide (CO_2)
Oxygen (O_2)
Alveolus membrane

Digestive system

Food entering the stomach may remain there for up to four hours. It usually takes about a day to pass through the digestive system as a whole.

Absorption of food occurs mainly in the narrow part of the intestine. This is filled with many small finger-like structures (villi) that give a large internal surface area lined with cells that absorb the products of digestion and transfer them into the bloodstream.

Section of small intestine

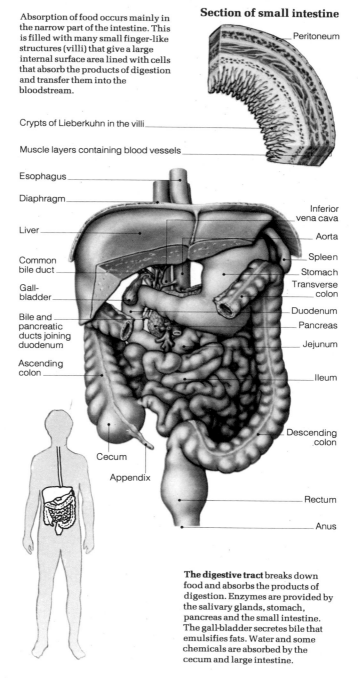

Peritoneum

Crypts of Lieberkuhn in the villi

Muscle layers containing blood vessels

Esophagus

Diaphragm

Liver

Common bile duct

Gall-bladder

Bile and pancreatic ducts joining duodenum

Ascending colon

Cecum

Appendix

Inferior vena cava

Aorta

Spleen

Stomach

Transverse colon

Duodenum

Pancreas

Jejunum

Ileum

Descending colon

Rectum

Anus

The digestive tract breaks down food and absorbs the products of digestion. Enzymes are provided by the salivary glands, stomach, pancreas and the small intestine. The gall-bladder secretes bile that emulsifies fats. Water and some chemicals are absorbed by the cecum and large intestine.

Urinary system

Blood is filtered through the kidneys, and excess fluid containing waste products and salts in solution (urine) collects in the bladder.

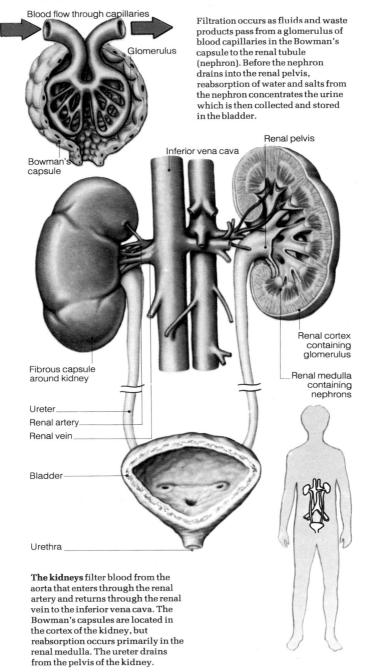

Blood flow through capillaries

Glomerulus

Bowman's capsule

Filtration occurs as fluids and waste products pass from a glomerulus of blood capillaries in the Bowman's capsule to the renal tubule (nephron). Before the nephron drains into the renal pelvis, reabsorption of water and salts from the nephron concentrates the urine which is then collected and stored in the bladder.

Inferior vena cava

Renal pelvis

Fibrous capsule around kidney

Renal cortex containing glomerulus

Renal medulla containing nephrons

Ureter

Renal artery

Renal vein

Bladder

Urethra

The kidneys filter blood from the aorta that enters through the renal artery and returns through the renal vein to the inferior vena cava. The Bowman's capsules are located in the cortex of the kidney, but reabsorption occurs primarily in the renal medulla. The ureter drains from the pelvis of the kidney.

Reproductive and endocrine systems

The main parts of the reproductive organs are illustrated.
Female organs are internal, whereas male organs lie both
inside and outside the pelvis.

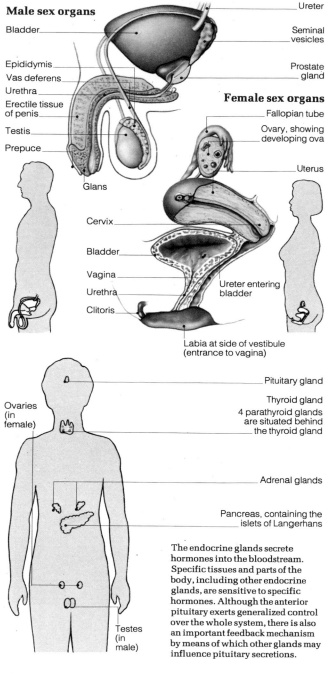

Male sex organs

Ureter

Bladder

Seminal
vesicles

Epididymis

Vas deferens

Urethra

Erectile tissue
of penis

Testis

Prepuce

Prostate
gland

Female sex organs

Fallopian tube

Ovary, showing
developing ova

Uterus

Glans

Cervix

Bladder

Vagina

Urethra

Clitoris

Ureter entering
bladder

Labia at side of vestibule
(entrance to vagina)

Pituitary gland

Thyroid gland
4 parathyroid glands
are situated behind
the thyroid gland

Ovaries
(in
female)

Adrenal glands

Pancreas, containing the
islets of Langerhans

The endocrine glands secrete
hormones into the bloodstream.
Specific tissues and parts of the
body, including other endocrine
glands, are sensitive to specific
hormones. Although the anterior
pituitary exerts generalized control
over the whole system, there is also
an important feedback mechanism
by means of which other glands may
influence pituitary secretions.

Testes
(in
male)

Symptoms: Charts of what to do

Introduction
These charts are a quick, easy way to help you reach a decision on what to do and when to call a doctor. They should be used in conjunction with the rest of the book. However, do remember that no book can ever replace professional medical advice: if you are still in doubt, or if your patient seems to worsen rapidly, you **must** contact your doctor at once.

Cross-references in italics in these charts are to the A-Z, and those in red to the FIRST AID section.

Contents

Backache	p.98
Chest pain	p.95
Constipation	p.92
Cough	p.96
Deafness	p.96
Diarrhea	p.93
Dizziness	p.91
Earache	p.94
Fever	p.94
Headache	p.97
Heavy periods	p.99
Increased urination	p.99
Painful joints	p.97
Painful periods	p.98
Rash	p.100
Sore or red eye	p.100
Sore throat	p.95
Stomach ache	p.92
Vomiting	p.93

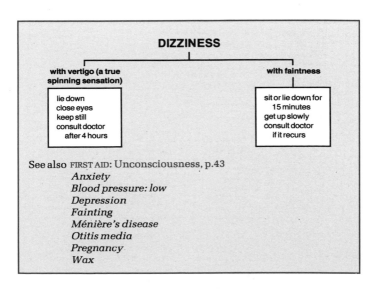

DIZZINESS

with vertigo (a true spinning sensation)

lie down
close eyes
keep still
consult doctor
after 4 hours

with faintness

sit or lie down for
15 minutes
get up slowly
consult doctor
if it recurs

See also FIRST AID: Unconsciousness, p.43
Anxiety
Blood pressure: low
Depression
Fainting
Ménière's disease
Otitis media
Pregnancy
Wax

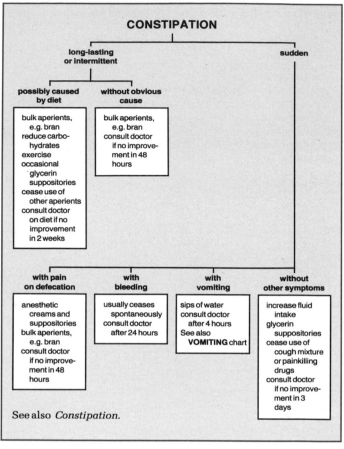

CONSTIPATION

long-lasting or intermittent   **sudden**

possibly caused by diet

bulk aperients, e.g. bran
reduce carbo-
hydrates
exercise
occasional
glycerin
suppositories
cease use of
other aperients
consult doctor
on diet if no
improvement
in 2 weeks

without obvious cause

bulk aperients, e.g. bran
consult doctor
if no improve-
ment in 48
hours

with pain on defecation

anesthetic
creams and
suppositories
bulk aperients, e.g. bran
consult doctor
if no improve-
ment in 48
hours

See also *Constipation.*

with bleeding

usually ceases
spontaneously
consult doctor
after 24 hours

with vomiting

sips of water
consult doctor
after 4 hours
See also
VOMITING chart

without other symptoms

increase fluid
intake
glycerin
suppositories
cease use of
cough mixture
or painkilling
drugs
consult doctor
if no improve-
ment in 3
days

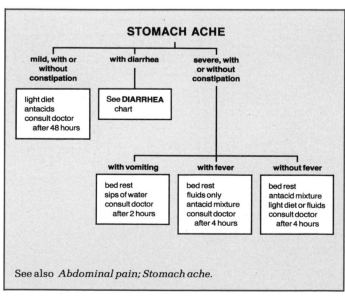

STOMACH ACHE

mild, with or without constipation

light diet
antacids
consult doctor
after 48 hours

with diarrhea

See **DIARRHEA** chart

severe, with or without constipation

with vomiting

bed rest
sips of water
consult doctor
after 2 hours

with fever

bed rest
fluids only
antacid mixture
consult doctor
after 4 hours

without fever

bed rest
antacid mixture
light diet or fluids
consult doctor
after 4 hours

See also *Abdominal pain; Stomach ache.*

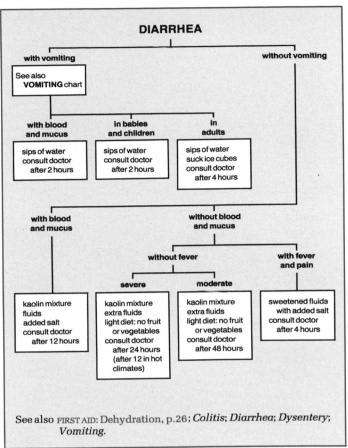

DIARRHEA

with vomiting

See also **VOMITING** chart

without vomiting

with blood and mucus

sips of water
consult doctor
after 2 hours

in babies and children

sips of water
consult doctor
after 2 hours

in adults

sips of water
suck ice cubes
consult doctor
after 4 hours

with blood and mucus

kaolin mixture
fluids
added salt
consult doctor
after 12 hours

without blood and mucus

without fever

severe

kaolin mixture
extra fluids
light diet: no fruit
or vegetables
consult doctor
after 24 hours
(after 12 in hot
climates)

moderate

kaolin mixture
extra fluids
light diet: no fruit
or vegetables
consult doctor
after 48 hours

with fever and pain

sweetened fluids
with added salt
consult doctor
after 4 hours

See also FIRST AID: Dehydration, p.26; *Colitis; Diarrhea; Dysentery; Vomiting.*

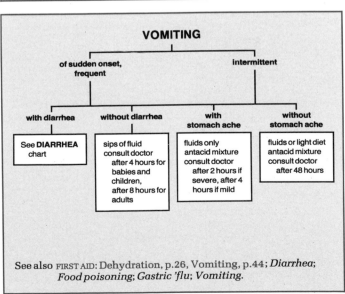

VOMITING

of sudden onset, frequent

with diarrhea

See **DIARRHEA** chart

without diarrhea

sips of fluid
consult doctor
after 4 hours for
babies and
children,
after 8 hours for
adults

intermittent

with stomach ache

fluids only
antacid mixture
consult doctor
after 2 hours if
severe, after 4
hours if mild

without stomach ache

fluids or light diet
antacid mixture
consult doctor
after 48 hours

See also FIRST AID: Dehydration, p.26, Vomiting, p.44; *Diarrhea; Food poisoning; Gastric 'flu; Vomiting.*

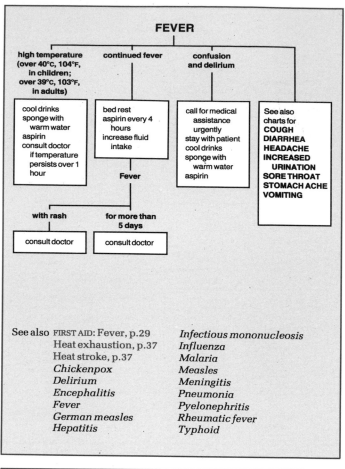

FEVER

high temperature
(over 40°C, 104°F,
in children;
over 39°C, 103°F,
in adults)

continued fever

**confusion
and delirium**

cool drinks
sponge with
warm water
aspirin
consult doctor
if temperature
persists over 1
hour

bed rest
aspirin every 4
hours
increase fluid
intake

Fever

call for medical
assistance
urgently
stay with patient
cool drinks
sponge with
warm water
aspirin

See also
charts for
**COUGH
DIARRHEA
HEADACHE
INCREASED
URINATION
SORE THROAT
STOMACH ACHE
VOMITING**

with rash

consult doctor

**for more than
5 days**

consult doctor

See also FIRST AID: Fever, p.29
Heat exhaustion, p.37
Heat stroke, p.37
*Chickenpox
Delirium
Encephalitis
Fever
German measles
Hepatitis*

*Infectious mononucleosis
Influenza
Malaria
Measles
Meningitis
Pneumonia
Pyelonephritis
Rheumatic fever
Typhoid*

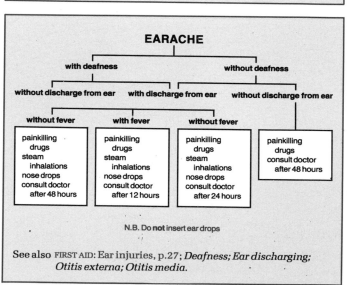

EARACHE

with deafness

without deafness

without discharge from ear

with discharge from ear

without discharge from ear

without fever

painkilling
drugs
steam
inhalations
nose drops
consult doctor
after 48 hours

with fever

painkilling
drugs
steam
inhalations
nose drops
consult doctor
after 12 hours

without fever

painkilling
drugs
steam
inhalations
nose drops
consult doctor
after 24 hours

painkilling
drugs
consult doctor
after 48 hours

N.B. Do **not** insert ear drops

See also FIRST AID: Ear injuries, p.27; *Deafness; Ear discharging;
Otitis externa; Otitis media.*

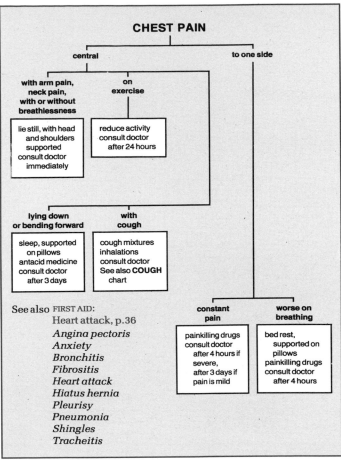

CHEST PAIN

central

to one side

with arm pain, neck pain, with or without breathlessness

on exercise

lie still, with head and shoulders supported consult doctor immediately

reduce activity consult doctor after 24 hours

lying down or bending forward

with cough

sleep, supported on pillows antacid medicine consult doctor after 3 days

cough mixtures inhalations consult doctor See also **COUGH** chart

See also FIRST AID:
Heart attack, p.36
Angina pectoris
Anxiety
Bronchitis
Fibrositis
Heart attack
Hiatus hernia
Pleurisy
Pneumonia
Shingles
Tracheitis

constant pain

worse on breathing

painkilling drugs consult doctor after 4 hours if severe, after 3 days if pain is mild

bed rest, supported on pillows painkilling drugs consult doctor after 4 hours

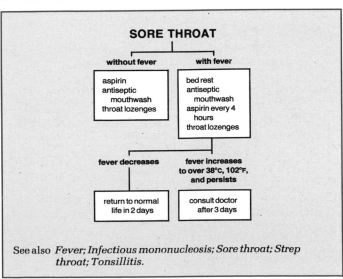

SORE THROAT

without fever

with fever

aspirin antiseptic mouthwash throat lozenges

bed rest antiseptic mouthwash aspirin every 4 hours throat lozenges

fever decreases

fever increases to over 38°C, 102°F, and persists

return to normal life in 2 days

consult doctor after 3 days

See also *Fever; Infectious mononucleosis; Sore throat; Strep throat; Tonsillitis.*

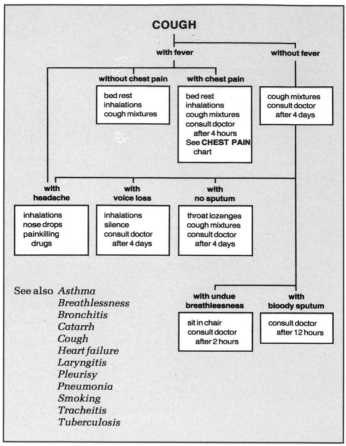

COUGH

with fever   **without fever**

without chest pain

bed rest
inhalations
cough mixtures

with chest pain

bed rest
inhalations
cough mixtures
consult doctor
after 4 hours
See **CHEST PAIN**
chart

cough mixtures
consult doctor
after 4 days

**with
headache**

inhalations
nose drops
painkilling
drugs

**with
voice loss**

inhalations
silence
consult doctor
after 4 days

**with
no sputum**

throat lozenges
cough mixtures
consult doctor
after 4 days

**with undue
breathlessness**

sit in chair
consult doctor
after 2 hours

**with
bloody sputum**

consult doctor
after 12 hours

See also *Asthma*
Breathlessness
Bronchitis
Catarrh
Cough
Heart failure
Laryngitis
Pleurisy
Pneumonia
Smoking
Tracheitis
Tuberculosis

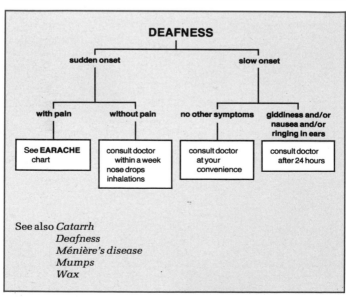

DEAFNESS

sudden onset   **slow onset**

with pain

See **EARACHE**
chart

without pain

consult doctor
within a week
nose drops
inhalations

no other symptoms

consult doctor
at your
convenience

**giddiness and/or
nausea and/or
ringing in ears**

consult doctor
after 24 hours

See also *Catarrh*
Deafness
Ménière's disease
Mumps
Wax

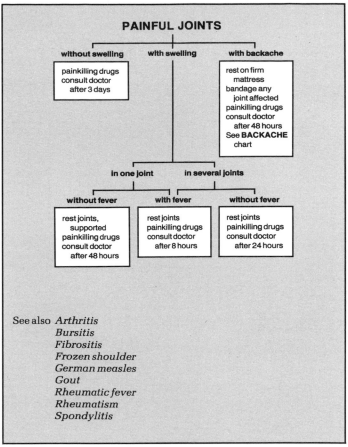

PAINFUL JOINTS

without swelling

painkilling drugs
consult doctor
after 3 days

with swelling

with backache

rest on firm
mattress
bandage any
joint affected
painkilling drugs
consult doctor
after 48 hours
See **BACKACHE**
chart

in one joint

in several joints

without fever

rest joints,
supported
painkilling drugs
consult doctor
after 48 hours

with fever

rest joints
painkilling drugs
consult doctor
after 8 hours

without fever

rest joints
painkilling drugs
consult doctor
after 24 hours

See also *Arthritis*
Bursitis
Fibrositis
Frozen shoulder
German measles
Gout
Rheumatic fever
Rheumatism
Spondylitis

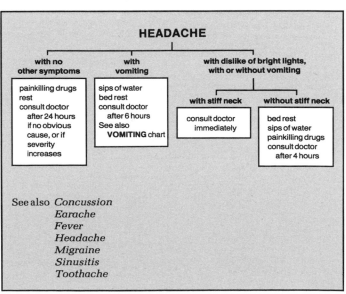

HEADACHE

**with no
other symptoms**

painkilling drugs
rest
consult doctor
after 24 hours
if no obvious
cause, or if
severity
increases

**with
vomiting**

sips of water
bed rest
consult doctor
after 6 hours
See also
VOMITING chart

**with dislike of bright lights,
with or without vomiting**

with stiff neck

consult doctor
immediately

without stiff neck

bed rest
sips of water
painkilling drugs
consult doctor
after 4 hours

See also *Concussion*
Earache
Fever
Headache
Migraine
Sinusitis
Toothache

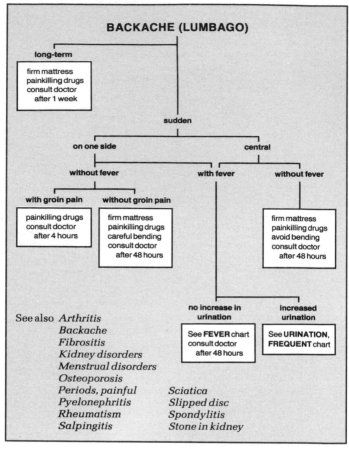

BACKACHE (LUMBAGO)

long-term

> firm mattress
> painkilling drugs
> consult doctor
> after 1 week

sudden

on one side — **central**

without fever | **with fever** | **without fever**

with groin pain

> painkilling drugs
> consult doctor
> after 4 hours

without groin pain

> firm mattress
> painkilling drugs
> careful bending
> consult doctor
> after 48 hours

(central, without fever)

> firm mattress
> painkilling drugs
> avoid bending
> consult doctor
> after 48 hours

no increase in urination

> See **FEVER** chart
> consult doctor
> after 48 hours

increased urination

> See **URINATION, FREQUENT** chart

See also *Arthritis*
Backache
Fibrositis
Kidney disorders
Menstrual disorders
Osteoporosis
Periods, painful   *Sciatica*
Pyelonephritis   *Slipped disc*
Rheumatism   *Spondylitis*
Salpingitis   *Stone in kidney*

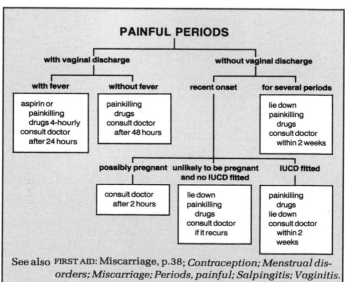

PAINFUL PERIODS

with vaginal discharge — **without vaginal discharge**

with fever | **without fever** | **recent onset** | **for several periods**

> aspirin or
> painkilling
> drugs 4-hourly
> consult doctor
> after 24 hours

> painkilling
> drugs
> consult doctor
> after 48 hours

> lie down
> painkilling
> drugs
> consult doctor
> within 2 weeks

possibly pregnant | **unlikely to be pregnant and no IUCD fitted** | **IUCD fitted**

> consult doctor
> after 2 hours

> lie down
> painkilling
> drugs
> consult doctor
> if it recurs

> painkilling
> drugs
> lie down
> consult doctor
> within 2
> weeks

See also FIRST AID: Miscarriage, p.38; *Contraception; Menstrual disorders; Miscarriage; Periods, painful; Salpingitis; Vaginitis.*

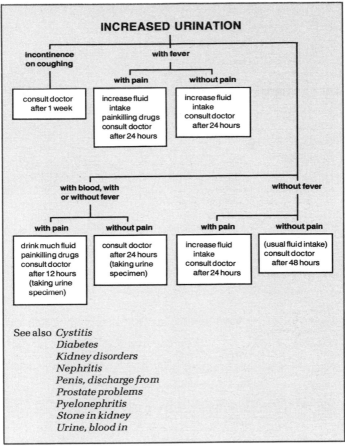

INCREASED URINATION

incontinence on coughing

with fever

with pain

without pain

consult doctor
after 1 week

increase fluid
intake
painkilling drugs
consult doctor
after 24 hours

increase fluid
intake
consult doctor
after 24 hours

**with blood, with
or without fever**

without fever

with pain

without pain

with pain

without pain

drink much fluid
painkilling drugs
consult doctor
after 12 hours
(taking urine
specimen)

consult doctor
after 24 hours
(taking urine
specimen)

increase fluid
intake
consult doctor
after 24 hours

(usual fluid intake)
consult doctor
after 48 hours

See also *Cystitis*
Diabetes
Kidney disorders
Nephritis
Penis, discharge from
Prostate problems
Pyelonephritis
Stone in kidney
Urine, blood in

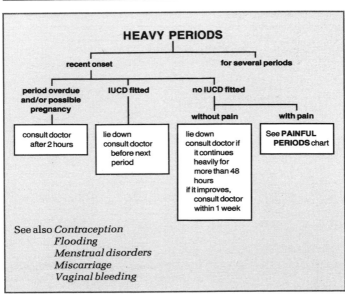

HEAVY PERIODS

recent onset

for several periods

**period overdue
and/or possible
pregnancy**

IUCD fitted

no IUCD fitted

without pain

with pain

consult doctor
after 2 hours

lie down
consult doctor
before next
period

lie down
consult doctor if
it continues
heavily for
more than 48
hours
if it improves,
consult doctor
within 1 week

See **PAINFUL
PERIODS** chart

See also *Contraception*
Flooding
Menstrual disorders
Miscarriage
Vaginal bleeding

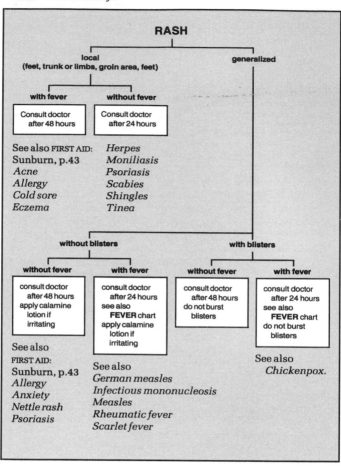

RASH

local
(feet, trunk or limbs, groin area, feet)

with fever

> Consult doctor
> after 48 hours

without fever

> Consult doctor
> after 24 hours

See also FIRST AID: *Herpes*
Sunburn, p.43   *Moniliasis*
Acne   *Psoriasis*
Allergy   *Scabies*
Cold sore   *Shingles*
Eczema   *Tinea*

generalized

without blisters

without fever

> consult doctor
> after 48 hours
> apply calamine
> lotion if
> irritating

See also
FIRST AID:
Sunburn, p.43
Allergy
Anxiety
Nettle rash
Psoriasis

with fever

> consult doctor
> after 24 hours
> see also
> **FEVER** chart
> apply calamine
> lotion if
> irritating

See also
German measles
Infectious mononucleosis
Measles
Rheumatic fever
Scarlet fever

with blisters

without fever

> consult doctor
> after 48 hours
> do not burst
> blisters

with fever

> consult doctor
> after 24 hours
> see also
> **FEVER** chart
> do not burst
> blisters

See also
Chickenpox.

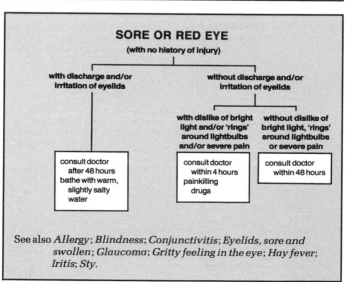

SORE OR RED EYE

(with no history of injury)

**with discharge and/or
irritation of eyelids**

**without discharge and/or
irritation of eyelids**

**with dislike of bright
light and/or 'rings'
around lightbulbs
and/or severe pain**

**without dislike of
bright light, 'rings'
around lightbulbs
or severe pain**

> consult doctor
> after 48 hours
> bathe with warm,
> slightly salty
> water

> consult doctor
> within 4 hours
> painkilling
> drugs

> consult doctor
> within 48 hours

See also *Allergy; Blindness; Conjunctivitis; Eyelids, sore and
swollen; Glaucoma; Gritty feeling in the eye; Hay fever;
Iritis; Sty.*

A–Z of diseases, symptoms and treatments

Introduction
This section is arranged in alphabetical order for easy access. Some of the entries give a full account of conditions that you may have dealt with, using the FIRST AID section, in an emergency. Many of the entries explain common problems about which you may want to know more, and there are also entries on some rarer ones that may concern you.

When to seek medical advice
Not all problems need medical advice, but if simple treatments do not work you should consult your doctor at a convenient time, by telephone or by visiting his office. If it is necessary, ask for a home visit by telephoning your doctor *before* 10 am. More serious illnesses need to be reported to a doctor at once, and emergencies require urgent medical attention. Such situations are indicated in the text by the following symbols:

H Call an ambulance or go to a hospital immediately.

☎ Telephone a doctor for advice as soon as possible.

Cross-references
In this section, a word printed in italics refers to another alphabetical entry in the A–Z. For example, in the entry on **Ankylosis**, "...degenerative changes in the spine due to *arthritis*...." indicates that you can also turn to the separate entry on **Arthritis** for further information.

Other references are made to the FIRST AID section and to the CHARTS OF WHAT TO DO, with titles and page numbers given in all cases to help you find what you need quickly.

A

Abdominal pain. *Colic* in the lower abdomen may be severe
☎ enough to cause sweating and *vomiting*. Continuous pain, if accompanied by *fever* and abdominal tenderness, may be due to infection such as *appendicitis* or to gynecological infection. If it is accompanied by *backache* and pain, with frequent *urination*, kidney infection may be suspected. A doctor must be called if it lasts more than four hours. If continuous abdominal pain is less severe, without fever, but is associated with *nausea, diarrhea* or *vomiting*, it may be due to *gastric 'flu*. Recurrent pain may be caused by an *ulcer*. Pain from an ulcer is relieved by food, but it returns later as a dull, central abdominal ache. Conditions such as painful *periods* and *colitis* will also cause abdominal pain.
TREATMENT. Medicines for indigestion will often give some relief but a doctor should be consulted for the correct diagnosis and treatment. See also FIRST AID: Abdominal pain, p.19.

Abortion. A term commonly used to refer to the deliberate termination of a *pregnancy*. The term is used medically to describe a

spontaneous abortion that occurs before the 28th week of
pregnancy. Deliberate abortions are sometimes performed as a
form of birth control. In some cases this method is the woman's
choice; in others continuation of the pregnancy would en-
danger the life and health of the mother. An abortion can be
performed using a special suction apparatus if a menstrual
period is overdue and during the first three months of pregnancy, or by a simple operation of dilatation and curettage (*D and
C*). After this stage prostaglandins may be used to induce
uterine contractions resembling those of labour. Certain cases
may require an abdominal operation. See also *Miscarriage.*

Abscess (boil, carbuncle, furuncle). A tissue infection in which pus
forms. A boil or furuncle is an infection of a sweat gland or hair
follicle, and a carbuncle is a large abscess, or boil, with several
openings.
TREATMENT. A small boil can be treated with local heat, from a
warm compress or a heated spoon, at regular intervals until the
boil bursts, when a dry dressing should be applied. A large boil
or abscess should be covered with a dry dressing and seen by a
doctor as soon as possible because it may require treatment
with antibiotics. See also *Breast problems: Abscess.*

Achilles' tendon. The tendon from the heel to the muscle of the
calf. This may rupture, particularly in the middle-aged, because of sudden strain on it when running or jumping. When
this occurs there is a severe pain at the back of the ankle,
accompanied by an inability to stand on tiptoe.
TREATMENT. An operation is required to repair the tendon. In
certain cases the injury is allowed to heal in a cast without an
operation but this risks leaving the patient with a permanently
weak ankle.

Acne. A chronic skin condition of the face and shoulders. It is most
common in adolescence, and is probably caused by a combination of factors, including the type of skin and hormonal
stimulus of puberty. Sweat glands are more easily blocked if
the skin is greasy, forming blackheads (comedos), the typical
spots of acne. Bacteria may infect the blocked gland so that it
becomes inflamed. Occasionally acne can lead to recurrent
abscess formation and leave *scars.*
TREATMENT. A healthy diet, avoiding sweets and rich or spicy
foods, and taking regular exercise in the open air may prevent
serious acne. Do not squeeze the spots, as this spreads any
infection. Wash the hair regularly, two or three times a week.
Wash the face, fingernails and hands several times a day. If
these simple measures fail, consult a doctor.

Adenoids. Pads of lymphatic tissue at the back of the nasal passages. Infection causes them to swell, leading to symptoms
such as *catarrh* and *snoring* and to secondary disorders such as
middle ear infections (*otitis media*) and *deafness.*
TREATMENT. Nose drops, antihistamines or antibiotics may be
prescribed. Recurrent infections benefit from the surgical removal of the adenoids (adenoidectomy).

A.I.D.S. (Acquired Immune Deficiency Syndrome). A rare new
disease, first reported in 1979. Most frequent among male
homosexuals and drug addicts, but also found in those who
have had blood transfusions from infected people, or who
come from Haiti. Probably takes about two years to develop, by

which time the body's immune system is damaged. Symptoms of *fever*, with lymph gland enlargement, often ending in death. There is no definite curative treatment at present. This disease causes great *anxiety* among homosexuals.

Alcoholism. The compulsive need for alcohol. Some people who depend on alcohol drink steadily and others have occasional heavy drinking bouts that continue for several days. Symptoms that indicate alcoholism include increasing inefficiency, aggressiveness, *polyneuritis*, and the deterioration of personal and family relationships. Further complications include vitamin deficiency, *cirrhosis* of the liver, *gastritis, convulsions* and *delirium tremens.*
TREATMENT. Treatment is effective only when the patient really wants to be cured. A "drying out" period is required with sedation to avoid the hazards of delirium tremens. Continued help from a psychiatrist or from Alcoholics Anonymous may help to maintain stability.

Allergy. A state of unusual physical sensitivity to certain substances. Allergies can occur only when the body has encountered the allergenic substance before. An extremely severe allergic reaction is known as *anaphylaxis.*
TREATMENT. Symptoms may be controlled by antihistamines, by cromoglycate preparations, and sometimes by corticosteroid drugs. See also FIRST AID: Allergic reaction, p.19·

Altitude sickness (mountain sickness). The reaction of the body to a reduction of the oxygen content of the air at high altitudes. This occurs most commonly during rapid ascent to more than 2,500 metres (8,000 feet) although some people are not affected below 4,000 metres (13,000 feet). Symptoms include *headache, breathlessness, palpitations, nausea, diarrhea* and extreme weakness.
TREATMENT. In mild cases, rest until the symptoms disappear. More severe cases require treatment with oxygen and diuretics and a return to lower altitudes. Patients with heart or lung disease should seek medical advice before ascending to high altitudes. Modern airplanes are pressurized to the equivalent of 1,500 metres (5,000 feet) so that there is no risk when they carry passengers at high altitudes.

Anal problems:
 Abscess. A region of infected tissue in the anus caused by local infection, perhaps from fissure-in-ano (see below), *tuberculosis* or, occasionally, *cancer.* Symptoms include swelling and severely throbbing local pain made worse by defecation. Sometimes bleeding and discharge through a *fistula* occur.
 TREATMENT. An operation is required, under general anesthesia, to drain the abscess. Careful attention with antiseptic dressings usually leads to rapid healing.
 Bleeding. The painless loss of bright red blood is usually due to *hemorrhoids* but may also be caused by *diverticulitis, intussusception,* an inflammatory disease such as ulcerative *colitis, cancer* or a benign *tumour.* Dark gray or black blood (melena) usually comes from higher in the digestive tract, often from a stomach *ulcer.* Painful bleeding usually indicates an abscess (see above), fissure-in-ano (see below) or a *fistula.*
 TREATMENT. It is important to consult a doctor. A special instrument (a proctoscope or a sigmoidoscope) may be used to examine the intestine, or the intestine may be studied by

means of X-rays following a barium enema.

Fissure-in-ano. A crack in the skin of the anus which may occur after *constipation*. It is painful and often causes bleeding on defecation. It is not uncommon in babies and in the elderly.

TREATMENT. **1.** Local anesthetic ointments or suppositories applied before defecation. **2.** Lubricants and roughage in the diet to produce large, soft stools. **3.** Sometimes an operation is required to stretch the anal muscle.

Itching. A sign of mild infection of the moist skin around the anus. It may be due to *hemorrhoids*, to a side-effect of antibiotic treatment or to infection with pin*worms*.

TREATMENT. Washing twice daily, careful drying and dusting with unscented talcum powder. Application of hemorrhoid cream may help, but if this fails consult a doctor.

Lump. Almost always a *hemorrhoid* protruding from the anus, but may also be due to an abscess (see above), a *polyp* of the rectum or a *prolapse* of the rectum (intestinal lining). In babies it may indicate a *prolapse* of the rectum, or an *intussusception* or warts (see *Verrucas and warts*).

Anaphylaxis. A very severe allergic reaction, usually to a drug or to an insect sting. The patient may feel faint, vomit and be incontinent, or collapse and become unconscious. Breathing may be difficult (wheezing). Extreme pallor is likely because of reduced blood pressure due to shock.

TREATMENT. Call a doctor or ambulance at once. An inhalation from the type of aerosol used by asthmatics can help. The doctor may give an injection of adrenalin and antihistamine. See also LIFE-SAVING: Checking for breathing and pulse, p.12

Anemia. A reduction in oxygen-carrying capacity of the blood. Mild symptoms are negligible but in more severe cases *paleness, breathlessness, palpitations* and fatigue may all occur.

TREATMENT. This depends on the cause but in most cases additional vitamins, iron and, rarely, corticosteroid drugs may be required. If anemia is caused by severe bleeding from post-operative hemorrhage, from a wound, or from a bleeding stomach *ulcer*, rapid emergency treatment is required. In less severe cases, caused by recurrent *nosebleeds* or heavy *periods*, the cause should be treated and iron tablets should be taken.

Inadequate production of oxygen-carrying red blood cells may be due to nutritional deficiencies of iron, vitamin B_{12} (the lack of which causes pernicious anemia), folic acid, vitamin C, or trace elements such as copper or cobalt.

Rapid destruction of red blood cells (hemolytic anemia) may occur in *malaria* and in adverse reactions to some drugs, or when the red blood cells are unusually fragile from a congenital fault, as in sickle-cell anemia and thalassemia.

Angina pectoris. Angina pectoris is a pain in the chest caused by lack of oxygen reaching the heart muscle. It is usually brought on by exercise. Typical symptoms include a constricting pain in the centre of the chest which may spread to the neck and jaw, to the shoulders, and down one or both arms to the hand. It is sometimes accompanied by breathlessness, faintness or sweating. It disappears with rest.

TREATMENT. Specific drugs to relieve pain and to dilate blood vessels may be prescribed. Angina pectoris is often a sign of heart disease but it does not invariably lead to a *heart attack* and care with diet and exercise may do much to prevent the development of heart disease if it is present. New surgical skills make it possible to replace the narrowed arteries after special tests. See also CHART OF WHAT TO DO: Chest pain, p.95.

Ankylosis. Ankylosis is the stiffening or fixation of a joint due to disease or injury. The more extreme "bony" (or "true") ankylosis is the fusion of the two bones that form the joint. *Spondylosis* is a general term for ankylosis of a vertebral joint or degenerative changes in the spine due to *arthritis*. *Spondylitis* specifically refers to inflammation of the vertebrae, and ankylosing spondylitis is arthritis of the spine.

Anorexia nervosa. A loss of appetite for food that cannot be explained by any physical disease but is attributed to *depression*. It is most common in teenage girls. The symptoms include loss of weight, sometimes vomiting after a meal, and often the cessation of periods (amenorrhea). A person suffering from anorexia nervosa remains cheerful and active and usually denies that there is any problem.

TREATMENT. Skilled medical advice and often hospital admission are required. Antidepressant and tranquillizing drugs may help, but treatment takes a long time and requires the co-operation of the family as well as the patient.

Anxiety. A common state of mind, often associated with a realistic assessment of difficulties, that may lead to physical symptoms such as sweating, *palpitations*, trembling, *insomnia*, lassitude, loss of weight and irritability. If a person suffers from *depression*, problems will seem greater and more difficult to cope with and so the anxiety will increase. Sometimes the symptoms of anxiety hide those of depression.

TREATMENT. May be difficult if the anxiety has a rational basis. Daytime tranquillizers and mild sedatives at night may help for a short time, but reassurance and moral support are of greater value than drugs. Specific therapy is likely to be most useful if anxiety is associated with depression. If antidepressant drugs remove the symptoms of depression, the problems causing the anxiety may appear less serious.

Appendicitis. An acute infection of the appendix, a blind-ended finger-like branch of the large intestine in the lower right part

H

of the abdomen. The cause of appendicitis is uncertain. The typical symptoms are *abdominal pain* around the navel which later shifts to the lower right abdomen, *nausea*, sometimes *vomiting*, and a slight *fever*, all of which develop over a few hours. The patient feels definite tenderness and pain when the abdomen is pressed.

TREATMENT. Consult a doctor immediately, and see also *Abdominal pain*. Surgical removal (appendectomy) is usually required as soon as possible.

Arteriosclerosis (hardening of the arteries). This is reduced elasticity of the artery due to thickening of the artery wall. It is made worse by high *blood pressure*, by high levels of cholesterol and fatty substances in the blood, by *smoking*, or by *diabetes*. Initially no symptoms are evident but the patient is in danger of suffering *thrombosis, heart attack, stroke* or *calf pain on walking*.

TREATMENT. Prevention is easier than cure. Regular exercise to the point of slight shortness of breath and a reduction of cholesterol levels in the blood by diet are necessary. Stopping *smoking*, reducing weight, and, occasionally, arterial surgery to replace a segment of a damaged artery, are also important in the control of this disease.

Arthritis. An inflammation of a joint. There are several distinct arthritic disorders. Osteoarthritis is the degeneration of a joint's surface due to age or to excessive use. Rheumatoid arthritis is a general disease of several joints marked by inflammation of the membranes and joint surfaces. The symptoms are increasing pain, swelling and disability over a number of years.
TREATMENT. Various antirheumatic drugs can be used, but aspirin in regular doses is the most helpful. Relief can be gained from regular muscle exercises and injections of corticosteroid drugs, although the latter may have serious side-effects. Devices to help the arthritic include special shoes for deformed feet and mechanical aids to help with dressing, washing and eating. Operations on the joints and, in some cases, joint-replacement surgery may be required. See also CHART OF WHAT TO DO: Painful joints, p.97.

Asthma. Asthma is a condition in which respiration is made difficult by spasms of the small breathing tubes (bronchioles). It is usually an inherited tendency that may be associated with *eczema* and *hay fever*, but it may also be due to infection, *cold* or *anxiety*. Complications include *bronchitis, pneumonia* and *emphysema*.
TREATMENT. Drugs may be used to cause the bronchioles to dilate. Some can be inhaled from special pressurized aerosols or sprays. Attacks may be prevented or stopped at an early stage by using bronchodilators or antihistamines, or by the regular use of corticosteroid aerosols or sodium cromoglycate inhalers. See FIRST AID: Asthma attack, p.20·

Astigmatism. Visual distortion of the shape of objects by a fault in the cornea or the lens of the eye. It can be corrected by wearing appropriate spectacles.

Athlete's foot. Athlete's foot (*tinea*) is a chronic fungal infection of the superficial skin of the foot, especially between the toes and on the soles. Symptoms include scaling, soreness, *itching*, and cracked and softened skin. The cracks may lead to inflammation of the underlying tissue. The condition is easily transmitted in public swimming baths, school gyms and other places where people walk barefoot. Careful drying between the toes is an effective method of preventing this fungal infection spreading.
TREATMENT: Antifungal preparations from a pharmacist may clear athlete's foot but if these do not work, consult a doctor.

Autism. A condition in which a person is totally absorbed in subjective thoughts that exclude and are not affected by the external world. In early childhood this failure in mental development prevents normal learning although it does not indicate low intelligence.
TREATMENT: This is difficult and only rarely successful.

B

Backache. This can be due to muscle, ligament, bone or nerve injury or it may be caused by an ailment in an underlying part, for example in *kidney disorders*. The sudden onset of backache is usually due to a pulled muscle (see FIRST AID: Pulled muscle, p.40) or ligament or, occasionally, to the *fracture* of part of a vertebra. Kidney infection (*pyelonephritis*) causes pain on one side with *fever* and frequent *urination*. Lung infections, such as *pleurisy*, cause pain in the back of the chest wall accompanied by fever and *cough*. Painful *periods* (dysmenorrhea) cause low central backache. See *Slipped disc*.

TREATMENT. Minor muscle and ligament injuries usually settle in a few days with rest and careful movement. More severe pain requires a doctor's examination. Pain-killing and muscle-relaxing drugs and sometimes an injection of local anesthetic often help. All such ailments require a doctor's diagnosis if they last for more than 24 hours. See also FIRST AID: Back injuries, p.20 and CHART OF WHAT TO DO: Backache, p.98.

Bad breath (halitosis). This may be caused by *smoking*; by infection of the nose, or of the gums and mouth (*gingivitis* and *gumboil*) or lungs; by tooth decay; by *sore throat*; by certain foods, fasting, stomach disorders, or *constipation*; or by general disease. Smoking is probably the commonest cause.

TREATMENT. The cause should be treated. Stop *smoking*, treat local mouth infections, clean the teeth regularly, and try to eat a light, easily digestible diet. Consult a doctor or dentist if the condition persists.

Bat ear. A slight congenital deformity that makes the outer ear stand out noticeably from the head.

TREATMENT. Cosmetic surgery, between the ages of four and six, may be performed if the appearance is worrying.

Bedsore. Ulceration of the skin on the buttocks, heels, elbows or shoulders in a bedridden patient. It is caused by lying in one position for too long. This restricts the blood supply to the affected area, which turns blue-black and ulcerates.

TREATMENT: Bedsores are prevented by regular movement, by rubbing the area with surgical spirit and powder, by keeping the skin dry, and by improving general health, with additional vitamins if necessary. Once a bedsore has formed there must be no further pressure on it and the area should be cleaned with an antiseptic solution.

Bedwetting (nocturnal enuresis). Bedwetting is common in children below the age of three. Most children are completely dry by the age of six but there are some who are still occasional bedwetters in their early teens. If bedwetting starts again some time after it originally ceased, there may be an infection, or an emotional cause such as *anxiety*.

TREATMENT. Wait for natural improvement. Offering careful encouragement, with charts showing which have been the dry nights, may also help.

Bell's palsy. An inflammation of the facial nerve. It causes *paralysis* of the muscles of facial expression and typically affects only one side of the face, causing the mouth and the eyelid to droop.

TREATMENT. Recovery is usually complete in a few weeks and may be helped by the use of corticosteroid drugs. In rare cases that do not improve an operation may be necessary.

Bent or curved back. If this occurs suddenly and is painful it is due to muscle spasm or spinal injury. See *Backache*. If onset is gradual, between the ages of 10 and 20, it needs specialist assessment and treatment. This is more common in girls and the cause is uncertain. If it occurs between the ages of 20 and 40 it is often due to bamboo spine (ankylosing *spondylitis*), which is a rheumatic condition causing deformity and stiffening of the spine, and requires specialist treatment. If it occurs after 40 years of age it is usually due to gradual loss of calcium from the vertebrae (*osteoporosis*) with gradual flattening of the bones leading to spinal deformity – the bent back of old age.

Birthmark. A blemish present at birth. Moles are common and seldom need treatment, but birthmarks on the legs and those that undergo sudden change in size or colour should be seen by a doctor. They can be removed by minor surgery.

Bleeding. See FIRST AID: Bleeding, p.21. See also *Anal problems: Bleeding* and *Vaginal* problems.

Blindness. The loss of clear vision in one or both eyes. There may still be an ability to recognize light and dark, and moving shadows. Sudden blindness in both eyes is very rare and usually follows an accident or a *stroke*. Sudden blindness in one eye indicates blockage of the artery to the eye from an *embolus* or a *thrombosis*, or a *detached retina*, or possibly an inflammation of the nerve, as in *multiple sclerosis* or *polyneuritis*. Momentary blindness may occur during the onset of *migraine*, or it may be caused by a small embolus passing through the artery to the eye. Low blood pressure at the moment of *fainting* may also cause momentary blindness (black-out). Gradual blindness may indicate *glaucoma*, a *cataract*, the degeneration of the retina, high *blood pressure*, *diabetes*, or recurrent ulcers of the outer surface of the eye.
TREATMENT. This depends on the cause and requires a thorough examination by a doctor to exclude general problems as well as specific eye diseases.

Blister. Blisters are caused by part of a shoe rubbing the skin of the foot and occur particularly as a result of long-distance marching or hiking. Not only the fluid-filled blister itself but also the surrounding skin is likely to be painful.
TREATMENT. Do not burst a blister, but keep it covered with a clean, protective pad. Harden the affected skin with surgical spirit and rest the foot if possible. See also FIRST AID: Blister, p.22

Blood, spitting of (hemoptysis). Any *cold* or minor respiratory infection may cause small blood vessels in the nose and throat to rupture, producing streaks of bright red blood in the sputum. This is normal and not serious. Infected gums (*gingivitis*) or teeth may also cause minor bleeding.
Bright red blood coughed up from the lungs may be a serious symptom but it is most commonly associated with *bronchitis*. If it occurs alone it may indicate lung scarring (bronchiectasis), *tuberculosis*, *cancer* of the lung or a blood clot (*embolus*) from elsewhere that has lodged in the lung.
TREATMENT. If the bleeding is serious a doctor must be consulted immediately so that the cause can be diagnosed.

Blood pressure:
 High blood pressure (hypertension). A common condition occurring with increasing frequency as people get older. Some

families tend to have higher blood pressures than others. Some diseases, such as *pyelonephritis* and other *kidney disorders*, are associated with high blood pressure. It will increase the likelihood of a *stroke, heart attack* and *arteriosclerosis*.

TREATMENT. As high blood pressure is often associated with *obesity* and *anxiety*, these should be treated initially and then, if necessary, a doctor will give blood pressure-reducing drugs.

Low blood pressure (hypotension). May be lower than normal following an illness, and increases the likelihood of *fainting*.

Blue baby. A newborn baby may have a slightly blue appearance. This is caused by poorly oxygenated blood in the circulation and is usually the result of difficulties in breathing immediately after birth. The blueness is apparent in the lips, the earlobes and the tips of the fingers. In certain cases the blueness does not disappear, and the tongue may also appear blue. This suggests a more serious defect in the respiratory system or in the heart. The hole-in-the-heart baby is a blue baby of this kind. Such defects must be repaired by surgery either at once or when the child is about one year old.

Body odour (bromhidrosis). Odour caused by the decomposition of dead skin cells and sweat by skin bacteria. It can be aggravated by *anxiety*, which increases sweating, or by a spiced diet.

TREATMENT. Daily bathing and change of underclothes are important. The use of antiperspirant and deodorant preparations may also help.

Bow-legs (genu varum). When babies start walking, between 12 and 18 months of age, there is an outward curvature of the legs. The legs gradually become straighter and even *knock-kneed* (genu valgum) at the age of about three years before they become naturally straight in the fourth year of life.

TREATMENT. There is not normally any need to treat this process as it will correct itself naturally. Rarely, bow-legs in a growing child are due to *rickets*. In such cases vitamin D supplements will strengthen the growing bone.

Breast examination. A woman should examine her breasts regularly, preferably at the same time each month. Stand in front of a mirror, raise both arms sideways and look at the shape of the breasts to see if any unusual dimples occur. Then lie on the back and feel each breast gently with the flat of the hand. The outer half of each breast will have to be felt by the opposite hand. Pinching the breast with the thumb and fingers will feel only normal breast tissue, whereas the flat of the hand will detect abnormalities situated within the normal breast structure. If any abnormality is found or if you are in any doubt, consult a doctor at once.

Breast problems:

Abscess. Breast abscesses usually occur during breast-feeding. They are caused by local infection, usually through the nipple, often because of a cracked nipple or lack of cleanliness. The symptoms are local pain, swelling and redness.

TREATMENT. Antibiotic treatment is required, with a doctor's prescription. In severe cases it may be necessary to undergo an operation to drain the abscess.

Babies' breasts. The breasts of newborn babies may sometimes produce milk. This occurs because milk-stimulating hormones from the mother's blood have passed into the baby's circulation and still remain to stimulate the baby's milk-secreting organs. This process will cease naturally within a few days.

Development. Breast development in adolescence is often associated with soreness. Most women have one breast slightly larger than the other and apparently uneven development is not abnormal. Approximately one adolescent boy in ten experiences tenderness in the breasts for a short period soon after puberty. Although this may cause anxiety, it is no more than a temporary effect and will disappear naturally.

Lump. A lump in the breast is not usually due to *cancer* but nevertheless it must be examined by a doctor. Various technical aids which include X-rays, mammography, and heat tests may help in making the correct diagnosis. It may be necessary to remove the lump for further examination with a microscope. Signs of cancer include puckering of the skin of the breast, red, weeping skin on the nipple and discharge from the nipple, some or all of which may be associated with a lump in the breast.

TREATMENT. If cancer is confirmed the breast may be removed (mastectomy) before further treatment with radiotherapy and with cancer-killing drugs (chemotherapy) is required. See also *Breast examination.*

Mastitis. An inflammation that may be caused by a breast abscess (see above) or by infection following nipple disease (see below). The chief symptom is soreness of the breast tissue, more painful than the tenderness that is associated with menstruation and breast development (see above). The breast will also appear red from the inflammation. It can occur during breast-feeding if the breast is infected through the nipple because of inadequate cleanliness. See also Tenderness (below).

TREATMENT. A doctor must be consulted. Antibiotic treatment may be necessary. Stop breast-feeding so that the infection is not passed on to the child.

Nipple disease. Sometimes a small amount of pale, milky fluid is produced during menstruation or when taking the *contraceptive* pill. Soreness of the nipple may occur when breast-feeding. Any other discharge or soreness must be reported to a doctor. If the skin of the nipple becomes red and appears moist without reason a doctor should also be consulted. Small sebaceous *cysts* may grow in the pigmented area of the nipple. These are not serious and can be removed.

Size. Breasts vary greatly in size and shape and the only definition of normal size or shape is that which is dictated by the fashion of the time. Nevertheless, breasts that are unusually large may cause discomfort as well as anxiety and breasts that are small may cause a feeling of a lack of femininity.

TREATMENT. In some cases, psychotherapy may help to alleviate anxiety. Cosmetic surgery to enlarge or to reduce breast size may also be considered, although it is expensive and is not guaranteed to be permanently effective.

Tenderness. Breast tenderness, swelling or tingling is common just before the time of the monthly period and in the first three months of *pregnancy.* If it is present for most of the month or if it is severe, consult a doctor. See also Mastitis (above).

Breath-holding attack. Such attacks usually occur between the ages of one and four. They are usually started by a sudden shock, accident or fit of temper. The child cries out and holds its breath for about 20 seconds, then turns blue in the face and falls down, apparently unconscious. Recovery time is about 15 seconds. These attacks resemble *epilepsy* but anger or fright at the onset indicate the difference.

TREATMENT. Ignore the attack if possible and do not give way to the child's temper. Patience and understanding are necessary until this condition improves naturally. Discuss the problem with a doctor.

Breathlessness. If this is acute and occurs for the first time it may be that something has been inhaled. Sudden breathlessness may be due to rupture of a lung, a blood clot (*embolus*), acute heart failure from a *heart attack* or an infection such as *croup* or *pneumonia*. Recurrent attacks of acute breathlessness are symptoms of *asthma, heart failure* or acute *anxiety*. Recent and gradual breathlessness may be due to a variety of causes such as *anemia, anxiety, asthma, cancer* of a lung or chronic *heart failure*. Persistent breathlessness occurs in *bronchitis* with *emphysema* and in lung diseases such as *pneumoconiosis*.

Bronchitis:
Acute. Indicated by the onset of a cough, often with thick sputum, and associated with pain behind the breast bone, *fever* and *malaise*. It often develops after a *cold*.

TREATMENT. Stop *smoking* and consult a doctor. Hot steam inhalations with menthol, a sedative cough mixture at night, an expectorant during the day, a warm room, a light diet and sufficient to drink will all help recovery. Antibiotics will be given if the doctor considers them necessary. The illness usually lasts less than a week if the patient is careful but a cough may continue for a further two weeks.

Chronic. *Asthma, smoking*, industrial pollution, *pneumoconiosis*, or repeated attacks of acute bronchitis will damage the lining of the breathing tubes (bronchi) and will prevent the normal drainage of mucus from the lungs. Because at night this drainage is slower, a morning *cough* to clear the sputum will generally occur. Coughing may also take place throughout the day. Recurring attacks of acute with chronic bronchitis need immediate antibiotic treatment.

TREATMENT. Stop *smoking* and avoid a polluted environment. Breathing exercises help to keep lungs clear of mucus.

Bunion. A bunion is a swelling over the side of the big toe joint, usually associated with a deformity which makes the toe point towards the other toes. Bunions are caused by tight-fitting pointed shoes, particularly those with high heels that throw the weight forwards. As the shoe rubs, the toe is twisted out of position and the skin thickens. A small fluid-containing area (bursa) forms in the tissue around the joint which swells to produce the bunion.

TREATMENT. In mild cases, it is sufficient to wear wide-toed, low-heeled shoes. If pain continues, a podiatrist should be consulted. The use of felt pads to separate the big toe from the others will prevent further pressure. In severe cases, in which there is considerable deformity and *arthritis* of the toe, an operation is needed.

Bursitis. Bursae are found at parts of the body where friction may occur, such as in the knee and elbow joints. They are pouch-like cavities lined with synovial membrane and filled with synovial fluid. Inflammation of a bursa is called bursitis and should be treated as *capsulitis* or *synovitis*. Housemaid's knee and tennis elbow are common examples of bursitis. See also *Bunion*.

C

Calf pain on walking. If this occurs regularly after mild exercise, such as walking, it is a symptom of poor blood supply. It may ☎ be due to *anemia* but is more commonly a symptom of *arteriosclerosis*. If it occurs suddenly a doctor should be consulted as soon as possible. It may indicate a pulled muscle (see FIRST AID: Pulled muscle, p.40) or, more seriously, a deep venous *thrombosis*.

TREATMENT. Consult a doctor for advice. If arteriosclerosis is the cause, stop *smoking*, reduce weight and avoid eating animal fats. A doctor may recommend drugs to dilate the blood vessels. Sometimes an operation is required to replace a diseased segment of artery.

Cancer. A condition in which the normal restrictions on cell growth in a particular area of the body are diminished or lost. Without these restrictions, cells grow to form a *tumour*. Local growth continues and cells may spread to other areas of the body through the lymphatic system and the blood. Tumours which grow at a distance from the original growth in this way are called metastatic tumours.

In many cases the exact cause of cancer is not known. Environmental causes, such as *smoking*, working in some chemical industries, and excessive sunlight (which may produce skin cancer, *melanoma* and *rodent ulcers*), are common. It is likely that some chemical substances in foods induce cancer and certain forms of cooking, such as frying in fat, may also encourage cancer formation. Virus infections produce cancer in animals and may cause some kinds of *leukemia* in man. Some diseases, such as ulcerative *colitis* and *cirrhosis*, may sometimes produce cancer in the area affected.

Cancer, in its early stages, is curable. The problem is to discover it before it has spread. This depends on the patient reporting to a doctor any change in the normal working of the body. The skin is easy to watch, and any mole or wart that changes colour or size must be shown to a doctor. A persistent *cough*, particularly in a smoker, needs a thorough assessment. The appearance of blood in the *urine*, a change in bowel habit and, in women, unusual *vaginal bleeding* around the time of the *menopause* may all be suspicious symptoms. A woman should examine her breasts for lumps monthly, after her period, with the flat of the hand (see *Breast examination*).

Later symptoms of cancer include loss of weight, general *malaise* and pain. These usually occur after the minor symptoms have been ignored but occasionally the cancer is so hidden that it does not cause any early symptoms and this is the reason why cancer diagnosis may be so difficult. Diagnosis of cancer requires the full facilities of a hospital. X-rays, blood tests and the removal of suspicious parts of a tumour for microscopic analysis may all be required before the diagnosis is confirmed and treatment is started.

TREATMENT. Cancer can be treated in various ways and often a combination of these must be used. Treatment may include an operation to remove the growth, X-ray treatment (radiotherapy) to destroy the tumour cells, and cancer-killing drugs (cytotoxic drugs) given by mouth or by injection. There are many kinds of cancer and so no single treatment can be used with success in all cases. Early diagnosis and treatment are most important, but the type of tumour, its location and the likelihood of rapid spread are also significant. Careful follow-up study ensures that any recurrence is found quickly so that further treatment can be given before damage is done. The treatment of cancer is improving each year. Anxiety should not prevent anyone seeking help, because what is feared as cancer is often something much less serious. Only a thorough examination will determine whether cancer is present or not and if it is dangerous. The sooner a diagnosis is made, the sooner treatment can begin.

Capsulitis. Inflammation of the fibrous tissue that encloses a synovial joint, particularly the shoulder joint (*frozen shoulder*). Capsulitis is usually caused by a strain or injury, and is indicated by pain and restriction of movement.
TREATMENT. The affected joint must be rested. Aspirin and antirheumatic drugs or possibly an injection of corticosteroid drugs into the capsule may be required.

Carpal tunnel syndrome. This is caused by the swelling of a ligament which presses on a nerve in the carpal tunnel of the wrist. The symptoms include tingling and sometimes weakness in the index and middle fingers and the thumb. The patient is liable to wake at night from the pain, and it can be aggravated by excessive use of the wrist which should be avoided. The syndrome is sometimes associated with *premenstrual tension*.
TREATMENT. Splinting the wrist and injections of corticosteroid drugs may help. An operation may be necessary to divide the ligament and so remove the pressure on the nerve.

Cartilage, torn. An injury to the cartilage of the knee. Each knee has two thin crescent-shaped pieces of cartilage which assist normal movement of the joint. A sudden twist or injury to the knee may tear the cartilage, causing sharp pain. The knee locks in one position or gives way.
TREATMENT. A large firm crepe bandage should be bound round the straightened knee. Pain-killing drugs are usually required. If symptoms continue, surgical removal of the cartilage may be necessary.

Cataract. An opacity that forms in the lens of the eye. At first it produces mistiness of vision but, ultimately, *blindness* may occur. A person may be born with a cataract, sometimes caused by the mother having *German measles* during the first 12 weeks of pregnancy. It commonly occurs in the elderly as a result of natural degeneration of the lens, and can be treated by removing the damaged lens and using special glasses or contact lenses, or an artificial lens inserted at the time of the operation.

Catarrh. Inflammation of the membranes of the nose with a thick mucus discharge. It may be caused by recurrent *colds*, vasomotor rhinitis, chronic *sinusitis*, nasal *polyps*, *allergy*, dust irritation, *smoking*, or a deviated nasal septum. In children it may be aggravated by enlarged *adenoids*.
TREATMENT. Direct this at the cause. Nose drops must not be used for more than five days as they may eventually irritate the nasal membranes. Antihistamines may help.

Chancre. An ulcer, the first sign of *syphilis*, that appears about
three weeks after catching the disease. It is a slightly raised
area with a depressed centre, but it is not tender. It occurs on
the penis, vulva, internally on the cervix, or occasionally on
the mouth. It will disappear in three to four weeks, leaving
only a small scar. Great care must be taken during the chancre
stage of syphilis because it is then highly contagious, and the
chancre itself contains the organisms of this disease.
TREATMENT. Cover with a dry dressing and consult a doctor
urgently.

Chancroid (soft sore). A highly infectious non-syphilitic ulcer,
common in tropical countries. A chancroid ulcer is tender and
yellow. Local lymph glands become inflamed, full of pus and
may discharge. The disease may affect the penis, urethra, vulva
and anus, and usually spreads rapidly.
TREATMENT. Consult a doctor immediately. This disease usually
responds well to treatment with antibiotics.

Chest, tightness in the. This describes a feeling similar to that
occurring after strenuous exercise. It may be a symptom of
respiratory illnesses, such as *asthma* or *pneumonia*, or it may
be caused by *anxiety* or *indigestion*. See also *Angina pectoris*
and CHART OF WHAT TO DO: Chest pain, p.95.

Chickenpox (varicella). Infection by a *herpes* zoster virus which
also causes *shingles*. The incubation period may be up to three
weeks and the patient is infectious for about two days before
the onset of the rash until six days after the rash first appears. A
period of three weeks' quarantine is required from the last time
of contact. The symptoms include fever followed two or three
days later by small red spots which develop into clear blisters,
then become milky in colour and form scabs after three or four
days. New spots may occur in the next three days and are often
preceded by a rise in temperature.
TREATMENT. Treat as for *fever*. A doctor may recommend antihistamine drugs and calamine lotion. Do not scratch the spots
as this can lead to infection and cause permanent scarring.
   Quarantine: 21 days after last contact with the infection.

Chilblain. Cold and damp conditions are liable to cause the hands,
fingers, feet and toes and sometimes the ears to become inflamed. The inflammation produces red swellings that may be
itchy and painful when the affected part becomes warm. Chilblains resemble a mild form of frostbite (see FIRST AID: Frostbite,
p.35) and if untreated the damaged tissue may ulcerate.
TREATMENT. Do not rub the chilblain but warm the area gradually. Pain-killing drugs may be used. In all but the mildest cases
consult a doctor. See also *Raynaud's phenomenon*.

Childbirth. The process by which a baby is born. Labour lasts eight
to 20 hours for the first baby and usually less for subsequent
births. Labour has three stages. The first is the longest stage,
lasting from the onset of labour to the moment when the neck
(cervix) of the uterus is fully open. In the second stage the baby
moves from the uterus through the pelvis. The second stage
includes the birth. The third stage lasts until the afterbirth is
expelled. The onset of labour is usually accompanied by backache, regular uterine contractions that become painful, and the
appearance of blood and mucus. At this stage the mother
should go to the hospital or call a doctor or midwife for skilled

medical care at home. The rupture of the amniotic membranes, with loss of the "waters," may occur at the onset of labour or later. See also FIRST AID: Childbirth, emergency, p.23.

Chloasma. A patchy brown pigmentation of the forehead and cheeks. It sometimes occurs during *pregnancy*, and may also result from taking the *contraceptive* pill or from disorders of the adrenal gland. In most cases it improves spontaneously. If it does not, or if it causes embarrassment, consult a doctor.

Cholera. A water-borne bacterial infection that occurs principally in the tropics. The first symptoms appear within five days of contracting the disease. Frequent, watery *diarrhea* and a slight *fever* are accompanied by violent *vomiting* and abdominal cramps. The greatest, potentially fatal, danger is from dehydration (see FIRST AID: Dehydration, p.26) leading to shock and circulatory failure.

TREATMENT. Antibiotics may help to reduce the diarrhea but intravenous replacement of fluids and salts lost through vomiting and diarrhea is essential. This must be performed in a hospital. Adequate sanitation, hygiene, immunization with a cholera vaccine and avoidance of unboiled water are necessary precautions for protection against cholera.

Quarantine: One week after contact with the disease.

Circulation problems. The body may be affected in a variety of ways because of problems with the circulation of blood. Abnormalities in the construction or dilatation of peripheral vessels may develop with age and result in the *dead fingers* and cyanosis of the extremities found often in the elderly. Similarly, poor general circulation may also cause *chilblains*, and a diminished circulation to the brain will cause a person to faint. The *blue baby* syndrome is caused by inadequate oxygenation of the tissues, and this may be a circulatory or a respiratory problem. Diseases such as *arteriosclerosis*, *phlebitis* and *varicose veins* also affect the general circulation and so may increase the likelihood of a person suffering a deep venous *thrombosis*, a *stroke* or *heart failure*.

TREATMENT. Specific conditions require particular treatments. To help prevent circulation problems as you grow older, stop *smoking*, lose weight and eat a balanced diet, avoiding saturated (animal) fats and too many carbohydrates and making sure of an adequate intake of vitamins and minerals. Take regular exercise, strenuous enough to cause short breath.

Circumcision. The surgical removal of all the foreskin of the penis. Medically this should be done if the foreskin is so tight that it restricts the normal flow of urine or if the underlying tip of the penis becomes recurrently inflamed (see *Foreskin, sore*). It is commonly done for social or cultural reasons. However, there are risks in this operation, particularly when there are bleeding disorders or the wound becomes infected. Rarely babies die.

Cirrhosis. A form of permanent scarring of the liver. Once it is present it cannot be removed. It is commonly caused by *alcoholism*, chronic *hepatitis* or severe prolonged nutritional disorders. Progressive cirrhosis may cause liver failure and internal bleeding leading to death.

Cold, common. Symptoms of a cold may be caused by any one of at least 40 different viruses. Colds are most infectious while they are developing. Symptoms include sneezing, *sore throat*, red eyes, general *malaise* and slight muscle aching, followed by a running nose for two or three days and then *catarrh* for a further week.

TREATMENT. Antihistamines, aspirin, throat lozenges and nasal sprays may help to control the symptoms. Stay in a warm atmosphere for the acute stage, preferably away from others to stop the spread of infection.

Cold sore. Recurrent blisters that break and form sores around the lips, often associated with a *cold* or *fever*. They are caused by a virus (*Herpes* simplex) that lives in the body and causes symptoms only when resistance is lowered.

TREATMENT. Immediate application of an antiviral preparation may be effective. Various proprietary lotions or tincture of benzoin compound may also help.

Colic. Colic describes the intermittent spasms of severe *abdominal pain* that may be due to intestinal obstruction, *gall-bladder* or *kidney* disease, particularly *stone in kidney*. Call a doctor if it lasts more than an hour.

In babies this is a sign of abdominal pain. The baby cries, draws up its knees and is clearly distressed. Colic is often due to *wind* and failure to get rid of it after a feed. Three-month colic commonly occurs in the evenings at this age and is probably due to a variety of causes such as a rushed evening feed, wind, boredom, or the change in diet as solids are introduced. It settles in time and may be helped by cuddling the baby or by giving an antispasm medicine obtained from a doctor. Colic may also indicate serious problems such as a *rupture*, a twisted bowel or *intussusception*, in which case the baby continues to cry and the pains obviously become more severe. A doctor must be consulted. In an older child colicky pain may result from the wrong food, *gastric 'flu* or possibly *appendicitis*.

Colitis. Colitis refers to two conditions, one mild and the other (ulcerative colitis) serious. The mild form is an inflammation of the large bowel (colon), producing intermittent *constipation* and *diarrhea* and sometimes *colic*. The causes are uncertain. Ulcerative colitis is a severe illness associated with *diarrhea* (often containing blood), *fever* and *abdominal pain* which rapidly leads to debility.

TREATMENT. Mild colitis is usually treated with antidiarrheal drugs and by increasing fibre and bulk in the diet. Ulcerative colitis usually requires hospital diagnosis and treatment with drugs and enemas. It is likely to recur and may require surgery to remove part or all of the colon. See also *Diverticulitis* and *Irritable bowel syndrome*.

Concussion. This term commonly refers to concussion of the brain, caused by a jarring blow to the head. It is often associated with temporary loss of consciousness, and vomiting may occur as consciousness returns. *Headache*, lack of concentration, irritability and loss of memory may accompany recovery.

TREATMENT. Treat as for shock initially – see FIRST AID: Concussion, p.25. Rest until all the symptoms have disappeared, with bed rest for the first 24 hours. It is important to avoid drinking alcohol. See also FIRST AID: Head injuries, p.36.

Conjunctivitis. An infection or inflammation of the clear tissue that covers the outer surface of the eye (the conjunctiva). Conjunctivitis causes watering from the eye, redness, and sometimes the discharge of pus with irritation and occasionally slight pain. Acute conjunctivitis often occurs with a *cold* or minor virus respiratory illness. More severe attacks are known as pink eye, caused by infectious bacteria that may develop into an epidemic in certain circumstances. Conjunctivitis also occurs with *measles* and *scarlet fever*. Chronic conjunctivitis is caused by irritation from dusty or polluted atmospheres and is often associated with *allergies*.

TREATMENT. Do not rub an infected eye as this is likely to transmit infection to the other eye. Do not wear a patch over the eye as this may increase the severity of the infection. Consult a doctor. See also *Eyelids, sore and swollen*.

Constipation. The inability to defecate because of hard feces. It is usually caused by slight dehydration, by a lack of sufficient fibre and bulk in the diet, by failure to open bowels regularly when needed or by excessive use of laxatives. Rarely it may be due to a serious physical problem, and a sudden change in bowel habit should be discussed with a doctor.

TREATMENT. Eat a balanced diet that includes fresh fruit and small amounts of bran. Fecal softeners and lubricants may be helpful, but avoid the regular use of purgatives. See also CHART OF WHAT TO DO: Constipation, p.92.

Constipation in children and babies. May be due to slight dehydration (see FIRST AID: Dehydration, p.26) or feeds that are too concentrated. Sometimes constipation is due to pain and bleeding on defecation (see *Anal problems: Fissure-in-ano*).

TREATMENT. Give extra fluid and, if the child is old enough, fruit and vegetables. A glycerin suppository or, in older children, milk of magnesia may be needed.

Contraception. Contraception prevents a pregnancy from occurring. Many different methods and devices are used but not all of these are equally effective.

Contraception for men. The sheath (condom) is an efficient form of contraception if properly used, preferably with spermicidal vaginal creams, foam or gels. Coitus interruptus (withdrawal before ejaculation) is not safe as sperm may have been produced during the earlier stages of intercourse. Vasectomy or male sterilization is a very safe form of contraception. It is a small operation, usually done under local anesthetic, in which the spermatic cord is cut and the ends tied. Vasectomy does not interfere with sex drive or ability and does not cause any physical side-effects, but the operation is a difficult one to reverse.

Contraceptive foams, creams and gels. Inserted into the vagina to kill the sperm. These are not safe by themselves although they may be used effectively with a diaphragm or sheath.

Contraceptive pill. Regarded as the most effective form of contraception. It is usually made from the synthetic equivalent of two hormones, estrogen and progesterone, or from the progesterone-like hormone by itself. It is a pill that is taken daily for three weeks of a four-week cycle. Menstruation usually occurs in the fourth week. Its main hazard is that it may cause thrombosis and this danger is greatly increased in those who smoke or have a history of previous *thrombosis, diabetes*, high *blood pressure*, liver disease (*cirrhosis*), *varicose veins*, *cancer* of the breast or *epilepsy*, and in those over the age of 35.

Failure to take the pill on one night should be rectified by taking two pills the following night. Missing more than one night means that protection is no longer effective and the packet should be thrown away and a new packet started after seven days without the pill. In such cases protection is not certain for the first 14 days of the new cycle. It is common for there to be no menstruation for six to eight weeks after stopping the pill and it is possible to become pregnant during this time. A doctor should be consulted if menstruation does not start.

Minor side-effects of the pill are commonly limited to slight *vaginal discharge*, occasional *nausea* in the first month and, rarely, slight weight gain. It very seldom causes loss of sex drive or *depression*. In most women the relief of knowing that sexual intercourse can take place without the fear of pregnancy gives a feeling of security and relaxation.

Diaphragm (Dutch cap). A special rubber cap designed to be placed over the entrance (cervix) to the womb to prevent sperm from entering. It does not harm the woman and cannot be felt by the man. If a diaphragm is properly used with spermicidal creams or jelly it is an effective form of contraception. Proper use of the diaphragm has to be learned and it must be fitted before intercourse and left in place for at least eight hours afterwards.

Intra-uterine contraceptive device (IUCD or IUD). A metal (copper or platinum) or plastic coil, ring or other shape that prevents the fertilized egg from settling in the lining of the womb. It is a safe form of contraception but it may cause painful, heavy menstruation (sometimes leading to *anemia*) or it may introduce infection.

"Rhythm method." A method of calculating the probable time of ovulation and avoiding intercourse at this time. It is not really safe because it only reduces the chances of pregnancy and does nothing positive to prevent it.

Sterilization. Sterilization of a woman is an effective means of contraception, but one that is difficult to reverse. The Fallopian tubes are cut and tied or clipped, either as an abdominal operation or by a technique using a special instrument (laparoscope) which can examine the abdominal contents through a small incision.

Convulsions and fits. Seizures characterized by violent muscular spasms that are frequently brief and recurrent. A convulsion may be long-lasting and violent or it may appear as little more than *fainting* accompanied by slight twitching. Convulsions may be a symptom of *epilepsy*, certain forms of poisoning, malnutrition, or of an illness such as *meningitis* or *tetanus* that affects the central nervous system.
TREATMENT. See FIRST AID: Convulsions and fits, p.25.

Corn. A concentric thickening of the skin on the toe or foot caused by a tight shoe. It is often tender.
TREATMENT. Protect the corn from further pressure with a circular corn pad. Corn-removing solutions soften the skin and so may allow the hard centre of the corn to drop out or be removed.

Cough. A noisy clearing of irritation from the respiratory passages. This may be from the throat and nose, commonly with a *cold*, *catarrh*, *sinusitis* and *sore throat*. It may also be due to problems within the chest from *smoking*, *bronchitis*, *pneumonia* and *heart failure*. Coughing is a useful and protective mechanism to get rid of infected or unwanted material.

TREATMENT. Many proprietary cough mixtures may help, while steam inhalations with deep breathing will help clear the respiratory passages. If a cough persists for more than two weeks or is accompanied by a fever, a doctor must be consulted. A persistent cough, particularly in someone who smokes, could be a sign of cancer of the lung. See also *Whooping cough* and CHART OF WHAT TO DO: Cough, p.96.

Cramp. A painful muscular spasm. This temporary spasm may be caused by a poor blood supply due to cold or a disease such as *arteriosclerosis*. Cramp may also be caused by insufficient salt in the diet to replace that lost by sweating, or by repetitive movements, as in writer's cramp.

TREATMENT. Warm, rub and stretch the cramped muscle. Increase the dietary intake of salt. Consult a doctor if the cramp persists. See also *Calf pain on walking*.

Croup. Croup is a harsh, barking cough combined with a rough, grating sound (stridor) that accompanies breathing. It is most common in small children in whom the respiratory tubes are narrow. Partial obstruction of a child's vocal cords can occur as a result of infection or inhalation of a foreign body. Croup also occurs in minor respiratory illnesses but is serious only if the child has difficulty breathing.

TREATMENT. A warm, humid atmosphere relieves the symptoms. Children also need reassurance. Antihistamines may help and breathing is easier if the child is propped up on pillows. It is often more alarming to parents than to the child, who is likely to fall asleep despite the rough breathing.

Crying. All babies cry. At first it is their only way of expressing themselves. They may cry for food, attention, because of discomfort, or because of pain from *colic*. Older babies may cry out of boredom. Let them watch you at work around the home and let them feel part of the family in the evening. Younger children cry because of frustration or temper, pain or fear.

Cyst, sebaceous (also known as a wen). Blockage of a grease gland may be followed by cyst formation if the gland continues to secrete. This happens more commonly in some people than in others. Symptoms include painless swelling just under the skin, most commonly on the scalp, at the back of the neck and on the shoulders. The size increases slowly over several years and occasionally may discharge a soft cheese-like material before continuing to swell.

TREATMENT. If it is unsightly or rubs against clothing, surgical removal (under local anesthetic) may be required.

Cystitis. An inflammation of the bladder. The infection may spread down the ureter from a kidney infection (*pyelonephritis*) or up the urethra from an infection such as *vaginitis* or *diarrhea*. Cystitis is much more common in women than in men because the female urethra is shorter. Symptoms include burning discomfort, urination disorders (see *Urination, frequent* and *Urine, blood in*), and *fever* in severe cases. Some attacks of recurrent cystitis are caused by sexual intercourse, because the massaging effect forces an infection into the bladder. This may be prevented by the woman emptying her bladder after intercourse and by careful washing. Recurring attacks of cystitis must be discussed with a doctor.

TREATMENT. Drink large amounts of fluid to dilute the urine. In more serious cases antibiotic, antispasm and pain-killing drugs may be prescribed. Local infections, such as *vaginitis* or skin problems, should also be treated.

D

D and C (dilatation and curettage). A simple operation, performed under general anesthetic, in which the neck (cervix) of the uterus is stretched open (dilated) sufficiently to admit a small instrument, a curette, into the uterus to scrape out the contents. D and C is usually performed to investigate *menstrual disorders*. See also *Abortion*.

Dead fingers. A sensation of numbness in the fingers often accompanied by stiffness. The cause is seldom serious unless there is a fracture of the elbow that obstructs the blood supply. An unusual sensitivity of the blood vessels to cold also causes numbness and paleness of the fingers. See also *Chilblains* and *Raynaud's phenomenon*.

Deafness. A difficulty with hearing that may be caused by blockage or damage to the outer or middle ear, or by damage to the nerve or the cochlea. A sudden onset of deafness is always alarming and until a doctor is consulted nose drops and steam inhalations may relieve middle ear blockage. Do not use ear drops. Sudden deafness and pain, with or without discharge, is usually caused by an infection of the outer tube to the eardrum (*otitis externa*), an infection of the middle ear (*otitis media*) or to sudden changes in atmospheric pressure. Sudden deafness without pain may be caused by *wax*, by blockage of the middle ear by *catarrh*, by a nerve infection following *mumps*, by a small hemorrhage into the cochlea, or by damage from extremely loud noise. A gradual onset of deafness is usually caused by *wax*, by repeated exposure to gunfire or noisy machinery, by aging, or by a family tendency to deafness such as otosclerosis (which affects the three small vibrating bones of the middle ear). Deafness at birth may be hereditary or the result of a maternal infection, such as *German measles*, during the first three months of pregnancy.

TREATMENT. In all cases, the earlier a diagnosis is made the better the chance of curing deafness and, in the young, of educating the child correctly and teaching it to speak in order to avoid dumbness.

Death. Death can only be certified by a doctor. If someone has just died suddenly or unexpectedly (e.g. drowning or heart attack), try and resuscitate them (see LIFE-SAVING: **Cardio-pulmonary resuscitation, p.16**) for at least 30 minutes.

What to do. If someone has just died, you must telephone the police and the doctor of record who will issue a certificate giving the cause of death, etc., which will permit clearance for burial. In the meantime, arrangements can be made for a funeral through an undertaker, who will register the death certificate with appropriate city and state agencies. If cremation is desired by the family, individual arrangements can be made with the funeral parlour. If the cause of death is not known, occurs unexpectedly or is the result of an accident in which someone else may be blamed, the coroner or medical examiner will have to be informed. He will issue the death certificate. There are many other things that need to be done following a death but your undertaker and lawyer will be able to advise you about these.

Violent death. If someone has been killed in a road accident or following a fall, or if you come across a dead body, do not move the body as this may disturb vital clues to the cause of death. You must inform the police at once.

Death abroad. Each country has its own regulations about certification of death. Do not move the dead person. Telephone for a doctor or the police and wait for their arrival. Get in touch with the local Consul (if the telephone book does not have the number, the police will be able to give it to you). The Consul will advise you on all the necessary arrangements.

Delirium. A condition in which the mental state is disturbed. It may be caused by medicinal or *drug abuse*, by high *fever*, or by infectious illnesses such as *typhoid* or *encephalitis*. Typical symptoms include excitement, thought disturbance, confusion and *insomnia*.

TREATMENT. Consult a doctor urgently. The correct treatment of the cause will shorten the illness.

Delirium tremens. A condition that occurs in *alcoholism*. It usually develops when the craving for alcohol is not satisfied and withdrawal symptoms set in. Hallucinations, sudden fears, muscle twitching, insomnia, periods of physical activity, and palpitations affect the patient for several days. Barbiturate addiction may also lead to delirium tremens.

TREATMENT. Admission to hospital for sedation and vitamin B injections is necessary. Recovery is gradual but usually complete after a long convalescence.

Depression. A sense of hopelessness and exhaustion that may follow any illness or treatment, or may occur without obvious cause. It may also be a result of grief or prolonged *anxiety*. Occasionally depression may be associated with periods of high excitement (*mania*) and it may be a symptom of *manic-depressive illness*. Typical symptoms of depression are lack of concentration, difficulty in making decisions, irritability, pessimism, undue fatigue, *insomnia, headache, anxiety*, loss of sex drive, tearfulness, suicidal thoughts and sometimes attempted suicide.

TREATMENT. Talking to a doctor about your problems is particularly important, because professional advice is usually the most valuable. Treatment with antidepressant drugs is common and admission to a hospital is sometimes necessary for severe cases that require psychiatric help.

Dermatitis. Inflammation of the skin. It may have a variety of causes such as an *allergy, anxiety, eczema*, or contact with irritating poisons or other chemicals, including certain cosmetics and detergents. Symptoms include redness, itching and sometimes other lesions such as *blisters*.

TREATMENT. Consult a doctor to determine the cause. Skin lotions may remove the inflammation.

Detached retina. Separation of the light-sensitive layer of nerves (retina) from the dark, pigmented layer behind (choroid). This most commonly happens after a blow to the eye or, spontaneously, in nearsighted people. There is a partial loss of vision with a cloud-like appearance, transient flashes of light and floating specks.

TREATMENT. Surgery, using laser or other techniques, to "stick" the retina back onto the choroid is very often successful.

Diabetes. A general name for two disorders characterized by excessive and frequent *urination*. Diabetes insipidus, a rare disorder in which the kidney fails to reabsorb water into the circulation, is caused either by a lack of the pituitary antidiuretic hormone or by a rare kidney abnormality. It usually responds to antidiuretic hormone replacement. Diabetes mellitus (sugar diabetes) is much commoner and occurs in two forms. The acute form, usually occurring in children and adolescents, may follow infection or appear spontaneously because of failure of the pancreas gland to make insulin. Diabetes of more gradual onset usually occurs in adult life and is caused by failure of the body tissue to react to insulin. This form is commoner in older people who are overweight and who have an inherited tendency to develop it. In *pregnancy*, women with diabetes or who have a tendency to develop diabetes will have heavier-than-average babies. Patients with diabetes for many years may develop *arteriosclerosis*, *gangrene*, *kidney disorders* and *blindness*. Very high blood sugar levels may cause diabetic (hyperglycemic) coma. It is of gradual onset, with drowsiness and deep breathing before loss of consciousness.
TREATMENT. Diabetes of acute onset requires insulin injections, while that of gradual onset may be controlled with a weight-reducing diet but may sometimes require drugs, or occasionally insulin. Insulin (hypoglycemic) coma (low blood sugar) is of sudden onset with sweating and palpitations. All diabetics, whether on drugs or insulin, should carry a bracelet or a card with their name, their dosage of insulin and what to do if they are found unconscious. See also FIRST AID: Diabetic emergencies, p.27.

Diaper rash. The chapping and chafing of a baby's buttocks and groin due to the dampness of wet diapers combined with the irritating effects of urine on the skin. It may also be associated with atopic *eczema* or with irritation of the skin by soap or detergent in the diapers. Occasionally *moniliasis* or an infection such as *impetigo* may occur.
TREATMENT. Always rinse diapers well and change them frequently. Leave the baby without diapers whenever possible. Zinc oxide and castor oil cream or a proprietary cream will clear mild rashes. Severe rashes should be seen by a doctor as antifungal treatment may be required.

Diarrhea. The frequent passing of fluid feces, which may be due to excess fruit, spices or rich food in the diet, too much alcohol, anxiety, *colitis*, *dysentery*, *gastric 'flu*, *diverticulitis*, *traveller's diarrhea*, *cholera*, or to the excessive use of laxatives. Diarrhea can be serious if accompanied by *vomiting* which will cause dehydration.
TREATMENT. Drink plenty of water. A kaolin mixture or antidiarrheal drugs may help. Before travelling abroad it is advisable to consult a doctor for a supply of drugs to control traveller's diarrhea. See also CHART OF WHAT TO DO: Diarrhea, p.93.

Diarrhea in babies. In babies this describes stools that are more fluid than usual. The yellow porridge-like stool of the breast-fed baby may occur once a day and that of the bottle-fed baby several times a day. Green stools are an indication that the intestinal contents have passed through more quickly than usual and the green bile has not had time to change colour. Diarrhea alone is not serious provided that the baby appears well and is eating and drinking normally. It may also be caused by an inappropriate diet. Dehydration may occur if the baby is not drinking enough or starts *vomiting* and this can be dangerous, especially in the very young. Diarrhea with *colic*, particularly if there is blood in the stool, requires urgent medical attention. See FIRST AID: **Dehydration, p.26**.

Diphtheria. An acute, highly contagious and often fatal bacterial infection that usually affects the mucous membranes of the throat. The symptoms develop after about two to seven days' incubation, and include severe *sore throat*, *fever*, and respiratory obstruction with patches of gray membrane in the throat. The toxin produced by the bacteria may cause *heart failure*, *palpitations*, and *polyneuritis*.
TREATMENT. An artifical opening in the windpipe (tracheostomy) may be required if breathing is very difficult. Treatment with a diphtheria antitoxin and antibiotics is essential, then slow convalescence with the strictest bed rest, particularly if the heart has been affected. The diphtheria membrane should not be interfered with unless it obstructs breathing.
Quarantine: Those who have been in contact with the disease should remain in quarantine until repeated throat cultures are negative. See *Immunization*.

Dislocation. A painful injury to a joint in which one or both surfaces are forced out of their normal position. Subluxation describes a partial or incomplete dislocation. The joint is unable to move and there may be obvious deformity. The victim should be treated initially as if the joint were fractured and should be taken to a hospital as soon as possible. See also FIRST AID: **Dislocations, p.27**.

Diverticulitis. An infection of little pouches that frequently form in the colon of middle-aged and elderly people. Often there are no symptoms, but *abdominal pain*, anal bleeding (see *Anal problems*) and sometimes *diarrhea* with *fever* can occur.
TREATMENT. A high-fibre diet, such as bran, and antispasmodic drugs will frequently help. If the symptoms persist or are severe, an operation to remove the diseased part of the colon may be necessary.

Drug abuse. The compulsive use of drugs due to a physical dependence on their effects and a psychological need for their continued use. The outlines of treatment for the main types of drug abuse are given below, but it should be remembered that each addict requires individual psychiatric assessment and medical care.
Stimulants. The most common stimulants are the amphetamines, cocaine, and others derived from these which are sometimes used alone and sometimes with other drugs such as barbiturates. Stimulants may be taken by mouth, sniffed or injected intravenously. Their effect is to cause a sudden increase of mental or physical activity, euphoria and loss of appetite. This usually leads to a confused mental state which may be accompanied by *paranoia*. Eventually there follows a deep sleep, followed by a period of physical lassitude and *depression*. A serious complication of sniffing cocaine is that this may cause perforation of the nasal membranes. Sedative drugs are required to treat stimulant abuse, together with

hospital care, followed by psychiatric assessment and therapy.

Depressants. The most common depressants include alcohol and barbiturates. Depressants are usually taken orally but are also sometimes injected intravenously. Mental confusion, slurred speech and unsteady walking are common effects. Withdrawal symptoms include *anxiety, insomnia, delirium,* tremors, *delirium tremens* and *convulsions.* Hospital admission is required to treat depressant abuse, followed by psychiatric care.

Opiates. The most common opiates are heroin, morphine and opium. They are sometimes inhaled but heroin and morphine are usually injected intravenously for rapid effect. First experiences produce *nausea, vomiting* and *anxiety.* Subsequent doses lead to a state of relaxation and contentment. Tolerance soon develops so that larger doses are required. Withdrawal can be acute with anxiety, irritability, sweating, sneezing, *abdominal pain,* vomiting, and occasionally seizures (see *Convulsions*). Admission to a special drug addiction unit is required to treat opiate addiction, so that sedative drugs and sometimes substitute drugs, such as methadone, can be used to relieve withdrawal symptoms.

Cannabis. The most common forms of cannabis are marijuana (leaves) and hashish (resin), prepared from the leaves and flowers of Cannabis sativa. Dried leaves may be smoked or the resin from the leaves used as an additive to tobacco or to food. Addiction is rare and is psychological rather than physical. The drug causes a mild drowsy state with an increased awareness of colour, sound and taste together with complex mood changes. Chronic users become apathetic, lethargic, and have difficulty in concentrating. Certain cases may benefit from psychiatric treatment.

Psychedelics. The most common psychedelics are LSD and mescaline. They promote an increased sense of perception, with images that fluctuate and change in apparently understandable sequences. The effect usually lasts about 12 hours, and occasionally can resemble a nightmare, when a psychotic or depressed state may result. Acute panic reactions or momentary recurrences of hallucinations may occur during the following few days, and these are likely to be the most dangerous aspect of the experience. An individual on a psychedelic "trip" should be accompanied to prevent physical harm. Occasionally admission to a hospital is required.

Miscellaneous. A variety of other substances are inhaled or sniffed for the physical or mental experience they give. These include amyl nitrite (a heart drug), nitrous oxide (laughing gas) and some organic solvents used in glues and nail varnishes. Such substances may have serious side-effects.

Dysentery. An inflammation of the digestive tract due to an infection from contaminated food and water. The symptoms include *diarrhea,* with blood and mucus, *fever* and *abdominal pain.* The infecting organisms may be bacterial or unicellular. Amebic dysentery is usually found only in tropical countries and may also infect the liver (*hepatitis*). Bacillary dysentery is caused by Shigella bacteria, and usually develops four or five days after infection.

TREATMENT. The feces must be examined, and antibiotic treatment follows an exact diagnosis. General care should be as for *diarrhea.* The feces must be examined again after treatment to ensure that the infection has been eliminated successfully. See also *Food poisoning.*

E

Earache. Pain in or just behind the ear. This is normally due to a boil or infection of the outer tube (*otitis externa*), to infection of the middle ear (*otitis media*), to *mastoiditis*, to pain from the jaw joint, or to pain that originates in and is referred from *toothache* or throat.

TREATMENT. Use pain-killing drugs such as aspirin. Do not use ear drops until you have received a doctor's advice.

Ear discharging. A discharge from the ear may indicate an infection of the outer tube of the ear (*otitis externa*), or it may come from an infected middle ear (*otitis media*), if the eardrum has ruptured. See FIRST AID: Ear injuries, p.27.

TREATMENT. Do not get the ear wet and do not use ear drops until you have received a doctor's advice.

Eczema. An itching skin eruption for which there is no external cause. It is related to allergic conditions such as *hay fever*, *nettle rash* and *asthma*. It may affect babies from about four months. Typically, a red, scaling rash appears on the scalp, spreads to the cheeks and to the limbs, particularly in front of the elbows and behind the knees. An intense *itching* causes scratching and insomnia. The condition varies greatly from time to time and may be aggravated by heat, cold and certain foods. *Measles* and *chickenpox* tend to be more severe than usual. Eczema may occur in adults, particularly if the person is under stress.

TREATMENT. During an attack, antihistamine drugs and corticosteroid creams may be used, following a doctor's advice. Cotton clothing and gloves worn at night to prevent scratching are advisable for young children. A normal diet is recommended unless an allergy to some food is suspected.

Embolus. A small blood clot, clump of cancer cells or other material carried in the circulation which may block an artery, causing conditions such as *stroke* or *gangrene*.

Emphysema. A serious reduction in the internal surface area of the lungs. This occurs because the small sponge-like structures (alveoli) that fill the lungs and provide the large internal surface area are damaged and collapse. This damage is usually caused by the coughing of chronic *bronchitis* and *asthma*. Emphysema causes *breathlessness* on exercise.

Encephalitis. A serious infection of the brain substance accompanied by high *fever* and dislike of bright lights, severe *headache* and *vomiting*. It requires urgent hospital admission and specialized treatment. A rare form of this condition – encephalitis lethargica – may progress to *Parkinson's disease*.

Epilepsy. Periodic and uncontrollable moments of confusion, loss of attention or unconsciousness. These may be accompanied by *fainting* or, in more severe cases, by *convulsions*. The cause of epilepsy is often not known.

Epilepsy is classified in two forms, known as petit mal and grand mal. Petit mal describes momentary loss of awareness lasting about a second. It is more common in children and attacks tend to diminish in frequency and severity with age. Grand mal attacks are typically preceded by strange sensations of smell, taste, and touch. The attack itself involves loss of consciousness and a stiffening of the limbs which lasts about 30 seconds. This is followed by rhythmical muscle contractions, often incontinence of urine, and sometimes guttural noises lasting for about a minute. The victim then lies unconscious, breathing heavily, for a few minutes before recovering sufficiently to move. Confusion and a severe headache may follow an attack, but these symptoms are not always noticed as the victim commonly falls into a deep sleep. Status epilepticus occurs when one grand mal fit continues into another.

TREATMENT. For treatment during an attack, see FIRST AID: **Convulsions and fits, p.25**. A person who suffers from epilepsy must be examined thoroughly by a doctor. Many antiepileptic drugs are available and most epileptics lead normal lives, despite restrictions against driving and against working with dangerous machinery or at unusual heights. A regular way of life and a diet that avoids alcohol are recommended.

Eyelids, sore and swollen. These may occur because of infection along the edge, blepharitis, or in association with *conjunctivitis* or *stys* and sometimes with cysts on the eyelid. It may also indicate excessive fatigue or be a reaction to a smoky atmosphere.

Eyelids, twitching. This commonly occurs on the outer side of the eyelid as an uncontrollable flickering (tic) of the muscles of the face. It is a symptom of *anxiety* or fatigue. It is not usually serious and should improve spontaneously. If it does not, a doctor should be consulted.

F

Fainting (syncope). Fainting is caused by a sudden drop in *blood pressure* which reduces the supply of blood to the brain and so causes a temporary loss of consciousness. Fainting may be associated with *fever, anemia, pregnancy*, fatigue, hunger, standing for a long time, some drugs, or bleeding following an injury. Slight giddiness, dry mouth, cold sweat, difficulty in seeing clearly, and nausea may all precede a faint and give sufficient warning that one should lie down or put one's head between one's knees. See FIRST AID: **Unconsciousness, p.43**.

False pains. Throughout *pregnancy* the uterus is gently contracting and relaxing. Towards the end of the pregnancy these irregular contractions become stronger and may cause *backache* and lower abdominal pains, resembling those of labour (see *Childbirth*), particularly at night.

TREATMENT. Mild pain-killing and sedative drugs may be required. Above all the woman needs reassurance that these pains really are "false."

Farsightedness (hypermetropia). This is indicated if there is excellent distance vision but difficulty with seeing close objects. It may cause *headaches* and watering, aching eyes when reading. It occurs as an inherited tendency, and can be corrected by glasses.

Fever. The normal body temperature varies with the time of day, within a range from 35.5°C (96°F) to 37°C (98.6°F) or even a little higher. The normal mouth temperature (37°C, 98.6°F) is often exceeded following physical activity, particularly in hot weather. Babies and children have a greater range of normal temperature. The temperature in the rectum is usually about 0.5°C (1°F) higher than in the mouth.

A fever is a temperature of 37.7°C (100°F) or higher that continues for more than four hours. Babies and children tend to have higher fevers than adults. Fever may be caused by almost any general infection of the body, and by some physical conditions. The sudden onset of a high temperature (40°C, 104°F) may be accompanied by a rigor (severe shivering) and followed by excessive sweating which is the chief means by which the body can lose heat. High fevers may be accompanied by confusion or *delirium*. In infants they can cause *convulsions*. Slight fevers are usually recognized before the temperature is measured by a sense of chill and general *malaise*.

TREATMENT. If the patient has a high temperature (40°C, 104°F) and is confused, *vomiting* or complaining of a severe *headache*, a doctor should be consulted at once. In other cases it is often best to use simple treatments and measure the temperature again in two or three hours. A fever is only one of the signs of illness and other symptoms should be taken into account. In all cases a doctor should be consulted if a fever persists. Simple treatments for a fever that can be carried out at home include soluble aspirin, bed rest, generous consumption of fluids, light diet, and cool sponging if the temperature rises above 39.4°C (103°F). See also FIRST AID: **Fever, p.29** and CHART OF WHAT TO DO: Fever, p.94.

Fibroid. A tumour of muscle cells that develops in the muscular wall of the uterus. More than one fibroid is usually found. Fibroids occur more commonly in childless women and only rarely become malignant. Symptoms include heavy *periods* and sometimes pressure on the bladder that causes frequent *urination*. Unless infected, they rarely cause pain.

TREATMENT. Nothing need be done unless the symptoms are troublesome or the fibroids are large. Individual fibroids can be removed (myomectomy) but others may grow later. Fibroids may disturb the lining of the uterus and prevent conception, so their removal is necessary if a woman wishes to become pregnant. Continued symptoms justify a hysterectomy (surgical removal of the womb).

Fibrositis. Inflammation of fibrous connective tissue most commonly associated with stiff and aching shoulders and back. It may be caused by over-exercise or by cold. See also *Rheumatism* and *Stiff neck*.

Fistula. An abnormal opening from a hollow body cavity to the surface, e.g. from the rectum to the skin outside the anus, or between two cavities, e.g. from the vagina to the bladder. A fistula may result from a wound, *abscess* or conditions such as ulcerative *colitis*.

TREATMENT. Kill the infection, but if the fistula remains an operation may be necessary.

Flat foot. A condition in which the whole surface of the sole of the foot is in contact with the ground, and in which the normal arch beneath the foot is lacking. The condition may be due to long periods of standing, to a congenital defect, to muscle weakness, or to *paralysis* following *poliomyelitis*. Children normally have flat feet for the first few years of life.

TREATMENT. If the foot does not develop normally exercises or a support for the sole may help.

Flatulence. This is caused by an excessive amount of gas or air in the stomach or in the lower intestines. It may be caused by air swallowing, partial intestinal obstruction, gaseous drinks, some foods, *indigestion, gall-bladder disease,* or *hiatus hernia. Anxiety* may also cause flatulence.

TREATMENT. The cause must be diagnosed and a doctor should be consulted if the condition becomes severe. In minor cases, indigestion medicines and regular exercise for those who live sedentary lives will be helpful. See also *Wind.*

Flooding. Profuse menstrual bleeding, usually so severe that it is difficult to absorb with external sanitary towels. It may be of brief duration or prolonged. It can recur with each period or it can occur unexpectedly between periods. Flooding is usually caused by hormonal disturbance, particularly a few years before the *menopause,* or by *anxiety.* It may also be associated with *fibroids, salpingitis,* or *miscarriage.*

Food poisoning. This is indicated by an acute attack of *diarrhea, vomiting* and stomach cramps, often affecting several people at the same time who have eaten the same infected food. It is usually caused by the toxins of staphylococcus bacteria, or of certain mushrooms or shellfish. In some cases organisms of the Salmonella group, which include the organisms causing *typhoid* and paratyphoid, infect cooked foods that have cooled. Botulism, a more serious form of food poisoning, occurs sometimes but is rare.

Symptoms of the onset of staphylococcal, mushroom or shellfish food poisoning appear within an hour or two of eating the infected food and include stomach pain, acute *diarrhea* and *vomiting.* The effect of Salmonella organisms that take time to grow on foods may not be felt for 12 to 24 hours but the symptoms tend to last longer. They are particulary severe in children and may be accompanied by *fever, headache* and general illness. Botulism is so severe and acute that immediate hospital treatment is necessary in order to save the life of the victim.

TREATMENT. An attack of food poisoning due to staphylococci or to toxins from mushrooms or shellfish is so abrupt that often it is over before a doctor arrives. The treatment is similar to that for *gastric 'flu.* A doctor must be consulted if diarrhea and vomiting continue for more than 12 hours, particularly in children. Antibiotics are not usually prescribed as the illness tends to improve naturally with the help of antidiarrheal drugs once the stomach is free from the poison. See also FIRST AID: Food poisoning, p.29.

Foreskin, sore (balanitis). This is common in babies and is associated with *diaper rash.* In adults it may occur in the uncircumcised due to poor hygiene or friction against wet clothing.

TREATMENT. Consult a doctor for the appropriate antiseptic or antibiotic treatment. *Circumcision* may be required if there is recurrent infection.

Fracture. General term for a broken bone. A fracture is described as being simple if the bone is broken cleanly with no external wound, and greenstick if only one side of the bone is cracked and the other side is bent. In a compound or open fracture the external wound extends to the fracture. A fracture is called comminuted if the bone is broken in more than one place. In a complicated fracture the bone damages nearby structures such as a nerve, artery or organ, and in an impacted one the bone ends are jammed together. A stress fracture is due to repeated minor injury, as may occur in a foot when running on hard ground, and a pathological fracture is due to a disease, such as *cancer*, that has weakened the bone. For treatment of fractures, see FIRST AID: Fractures, p.29 and Fractures and bandaging, p.30

Frozen shoulder. This describes a painful shoulder, the movement of which is restricted. It may be associated with *fibrositis*, *bursitis*, *capsulitis*, or sometimes with a heart attack or chest problem. Recovery may take a long time.
TREATMENT. Pain-killing and antirheumatic drugs, shortwave heat treatment and physiotherapy may help and an injection of corticosteroid drugs is sometimes effective.

G

Gall-bladder disease. The gall-bladder lies under the liver. It excretes unwanted substances such as cholesterol and bilirubin in the bile. The gall-bladder also stores bile and discharges it into the small intestine where it aids the digestion of fat. Gall-stones, consisting of a sediment of cholesterol, bilirubin and bile salts, may occur in those with excess cholesterol in the blood or as a result of an infection of the gall-bladder (cholecystitis). Symptoms of gall-stones include severe *abdominal pain*, *colic*, sweating and *vomiting*, or possibly *jaundice* due to blockage of the bile ducts by a gall-stone. Chronic gall-bladder disease may be associated with *colic* or with no clear symptoms apart from darker urine and paler stools than normal.
TREATMENT. Appropriate antibiotics and admission to a hospital are usually required to treat an acute attack of cholecystitis. Chronic infections will probably require an operation to remove the gall-bladder (cholecystectomy). About 20% of the population over the age of 60 have gall-stones. They need to be removed only if they cause adverse symptoms.

Gangrene. The death of an area of tissue that is still part of a living body. It is usually caused by blockage of the blood supply to the affected area. This may be the result of an accident, of severe *arteriosclerosis*, of infection, of *embolus*, or possibly of frostbite. Dry gangrene usually affects the extremities, particularly the toes or fingers. The tissues are seen to shrivel and darken. Sudden blockage of an artery leads to painful swelling of the area, which may then become infected. Infection, particularly if the blood supply is poor, may lead to infective gangrene, with black, wet, discharging tissue.
Gas gangrene is a severe form of infection in the tissues as a result of a wound. It is associated with the production of gas and poisons by bacteria in the infected tissue that can ultimately affect the whole body and cause death.
TREATMENT. Consult a doctor at once. Cover the area with a light, dry dressing. Do not warm the area. Admission to a hospital may be necessary for appropriate treatment with antibiotics and dressings to kill any infection. Sometimes an operation is required to improve the blood supply or amputate the limb. See also FIRST AID: Frostbite, p.35

Gastric 'flu. The term is used to describe the sudden onset of severe *vomiting* with or without *diarrhea*, *abdominal pain* and *colic*. Typically it starts during the night and lasts three to six hours. This is followed by a few hours of extreme *nausea*, with occasional vomiting or diarrhea before the onset of slight muscle aching, *headache* and sometimes a temperature of up to 37.8°C (100°F). The illness passes in 36 to 48 hours, leaving general *malaise* which lasts a further two days. It is caused by a virus infection (but not the influenza virus). The symptoms are similar to *food poisoning*.

TREATMENT. Do not attempt to drink anything until all vomiting has stopped, then start with sips of water and increase the quantity slowly. Ice cubes and mouth washes help. Call a doctor if the illness lasts more than 24 hours.

Gastritis. An inflammation of the stomach which may result from *smoking*, *alcoholism* or the wrong kind of diet. It also occurs with *gastric 'flu* and sometimes with *anxiety* and *depression*. The usual symptoms are *malaise*, *nausea*, and sometimes *vomiting* with *abdominal pain*.

TREATMENT. Stop any causative condition, such as *smoking*, and take regular small meals and antacids. If the symptoms persist consult your doctor.

German measles (rubella). A virus infection that causes a mild fever and *sore throat* for one or two days, followed by a fine, orange-pink *rash* on the face that spreads over the body. The rash lasts two or three days. Tender, swollen glands at the back of the head may last for about ten days. Adults with German measles may develop painful swollen joints of the limbs. The most serious complications of rubella affect the child born to a woman who has the disease during the first three months of pregnancy. *Cataracts*, congenital heart problems, *deafness*, and other abnormalities may be found in the baby.

TREATMENT. Treat as for *fever*. Lotions to soothe the itching may help. The patient must be isolated from any woman who might be in the early (undetected) stages of pregnancy or in the first three months of pregnancy.

Quarantine: 21 days after last contact with the disease. See also *Immunization*.

Gingivitis. An inflammation of the gums that starts around the teeth. The gums become swollen and tender and are likely to bleed. If it is not treated an infection around the teeth (periodontitis) may occur.

TREATMENT. Regular brushing of the teeth and a diet of food that needs chewing, without sugar and with plenty of vitamins, helps to prevent inflammation. Dental treatment of decayed teeth and regular scraping of tartar from the enamel is also necessary. See also *Gumboil* and *Toothache*.

Glaucoma. This is a condition in which the pressure of the fluid in the eye increases. This pressure prevents the normal circulation of blood, damages the nerve cells that respond to light and ultimately causes *blindness*. Symptoms are a gradual or intermittent deterioration of vision, rings or haloes around bright lights, a red eye and severe eye pain, sometimes accompanied by *vomiting*.

TREATMENT. Careful medical supervision is required to detect pressure changes in the eye. The acute, painful, red eye with blurred vision must be reported immediately to a doctor.

Glossitis. This inflammation results in a smooth, red, sometimes sore tongue. It may be due to the excessive use of antibiotics or other medicaments, or to a lack of *vitamins* of the B group. It may also be a symptom of pernicious *anemia.*

TREATMENT. Extra vitamin B should be given, and antiseptic mouth washes used sparingly. A doctor should be consulted if there is no improvement after a few days.

Gonorrhea. A contagious sexually transmitted bacterial infection of the genital mucous membranes of either sex. Inflammation appears within a week of contracting the disease. Gonorrhea may also affect other parts of the body such as the conjunctiva and oral mucosa, rectum or joints. In the male, gonorrhea may cause pain on urination and be detected by a milky discharge from the *penis.* Although the disease may not cause symptoms in the female, *cystitis, vaginal discharge* and tenderness are often present.

TREATMENT. Avoid further sexual intercourse and consult a doctor. Penicillin is the most effective treatment but occasionally the infecting bacteria are resistant and other antibiotics must be used. See also *Non-specific urethritis.*

Gout. A disorder of the body's metabolism (hyperuricemia) in which the normal disposal of uric acid is disrupted. As a result, salts of uric acid accumulate in the joints causing pain and inflammation. Ultimately gout may cause *arthritis* of the affected joints. It may also involve the kidneys where crystallized uric acid may be deposited. Attacks may be precipitated by a large meal, drinking alcohol, illness, an operation, an accident, or fatigue.

TREATMENT. An acute attack can be treated under medical supervision with large doses of antirheumatic drugs. Antigout drugs will help to prevent attacks by reducing the level of uric acid in the body. The pain is eased by rest with the affected joints raised. Massage and warmth from hot dressings may also give relief.

Granuloma inguinale. A sexually transmitted bacterial infection that is most common in tropical countries. The sign of infection is a small nodule in the genital area which slowly begins to ulcerate.

TREATMENT. Consult a doctor. Treatment with antibiotics is usually effective.

Gritty feeling in the eye. This is only rarely due to dust or a foreign body. Usually it is a symptom of *conjunctivitis.*

Gumboil. An abscess on the gum, usually caused by infection of a decayed tooth.

TREATMENT. Use pain-killing drugs, antiseptic mouth washes and gargles until the gumboil can be seen by a dentist or a doctor. Treatment with antibiotics may be required before the tooth decay can be dealt with. See FIRST AID: Dental problems, p.26.

H

Hay fever (allergic rhinitis). An *allergy* affecting the mucous air passages of the nose and throat. It is caused by grass or flower pollens, hay or house dust, and other external irritants. Pollen allergies are seasonal and tend to occur at the same time each year for the individual sufferer. Symptoms include catarrhal inflammation, a running nose, sneezing and watering eyes. *Asthma* may also occur.

TREATMENT. Inoculations with extracts of the particular allergen are sometimes successful. Antihistamines reduce symptoms but introduce problems, such as drowsiness, which may be unacceptable, especially at work, when using machinery or when driving. Anti-inflammatory nasal sprays control most symptoms.

Headache. This is a symptom, not a disorder. Possible causes of headache include *anxiety* and *depression*; *migraine*; pressure on the nerves supplying the scalp (neuralgia); many conditions, especially infections, such as *sinusitis, sore throat, meningitis, encephalitis* and those affecting the ears (*otitis media*); head injuries (see FIRST AID: Head injuries, p.36); and many other conditions.

TREATMENT. Most headaches respond well to pain-killing drugs, such as aspirin, and a good night's rest. However, as a headache is a symptom of so many disorders, a doctor should be consulted if it persists. Those who have severe headaches with fever, vomiting, neck stiffness and dislike of bright light should see a doctor urgently. See also CHART OF WHAT TO DO: Headache, p.97.

Heart attack. A lay term for a coronary thrombosis (myocardial infarction) caused by the blockage of a branch of a coronary artery. This blockage prevents oxygenated blood from reaching part of the heart muscle, and so affects the action of the heart. Typical symptoms include severe, constricting midchest pain that may spread to one or both shoulders, down the arms to the hands, up the neck to the jaw and into the upper abdomen. This pain is often accompanied by *nausea, vomiting* and sweating and may be followed by shock, due to the drop in blood pressure, and irregular pulse.

TREATMENT. For heart massage, see LIFE-SAVING: Heart massage, p.13. As the patient recovers from the heart attack bed rest at home or special nursing in a coronary-care unit in a hospital are required. Anticoagulant drugs may be given in certain cases. Following recovery the patient should take regular exercise, lose weight, stop smoking and reduce the proportion of animal fat in the diet. See also CHART OF WHAT TO DO: Chest pain, p.95.

Heartburn. A moderately painful, burning sensation occurring behind the breastbone and in the pit of the stomach. This has nothing to do with heart disease but is a type of *indigestion*. It is caused by a spasm of the lower end of the gullet (esophagus) aggravated by acid leaking back from the stomach. This may occur in *hiatus hernia*, after a large meal, when bending forward or after too much alcohol.

Heart failure. Failure of the heart to pump blood around the body in adequate amounts. Heart failure may be caused by heart valve disease, high *blood pressure*, or damage to heart muscle following a *heart attack*. Symptoms include *breathlessness*, ankle swelling, coughing and a bluish tinge to the lips.

TREATMENT. Careful medical treatment with heart and diuretic drugs is required in most cases, with bed rest and extra oxygen if this is needed to help breathing.

Heberden's nodes. Cartilaginous and bony nodules that occur near the end joints of mildly osteoarthritic fingers (see *Arthritis*), particularly in the elderly. Sometimes the nodules may be tender and inflamed but usually the inflammation settles without treatment in two or three weeks.

Hemorrhoids (piles). Dilated veins that occur inside or outside the ring of anal muscle. They are caused by *constipation, diarrhea*, pressure on local veins during *pregnancy* or, occasionally, by a tumour. Symptoms include bleeding, itching and soreness, with a protruding lump.
TREATMENT. **1.** Washing and careful drying of the area twice a day and regular defecation. If necessary, mild laxatives may be used. Additional fibre bulk in the diet assists the treatment. **2.** Ointments and suppositories may be used overnight. **3.** Anesthetic and antibiotic preparations are sometimes prescribed by a doctor. **4.** Injections may also be given deliberately to cause thrombosis (blood-clotting) of the piles and scarring, which produces minor discomfort and is usually done in the surgery. **5.** Anal muscle can be stretched under general anesthetic. **6.** Surgical removal of the piles (hemorrhoidectomy) is a more complicated operation and may require seven to ten days in hospital. See also *Anal problems* and FIRST AID: Hemorrhoids, p.37.

Hepatitis. A serious liver infection caused by a variety of viruses. It can sometimes be a complication of amebic *dysentery*, certain drugs or *alcoholism*. Infectious hepatitis is caused by various viruses (A, B, and non-A and non-B). Virus B, the most serious infection, is usually caught by blood transfusion, sexual intercourse or from shared needles used in *drug abuse*. The symptoms include weakness, *fever, nausea, jaundice* and *abdominal pain*.
TREATMENT. A doctor must be consulted and it may be necessary to admit the patient to a hospital. Anyone suffering from hepatitis must be particularly careful with diet and general health during the extended period of recovery. Plenty of rest and a diet that contains large amounts of fresh fruit and vegetables and avoids fat will speed recovery. Alcohol should not be drunk for six months. Care must be taken not to transmit the disease to others. All contacts should be given injections of gamma globulin. A vaccine against the virus B hepatitis is now available from your doctor: see *Immunization*.

Herpes. There are four distinct groups of herpes virus: **1.** Herpes simplex which causes *cold sores, herpes genitalis* and, rarely, *encephalitis*. **2.** A group of Cytomegalovirus which can cause an *infectious mononucleosis*-like illness and is a common cause of congenital deformity when it occurs in pregnant mothers. **3.** Epstein-Barr virus which may cause *infectious mononucleosis* and two rare forms of *cancer*. **4.** Varicella which produces *chickenpox* and *shingles*.

Herpes genitalis. A virus, causing an infection like a *cold sore* in the genital region. It is usually but not always transmitted through sexual intercourse. Symptoms include painful blisters in the genital region which become inflamed.
TREATMENT. After seven to ten days the sores will begin to disappear. Cold compresses, antiviral and pain-killing drugs may help. A doctor must be consulted.

Hiatus hernia. The diaphragm, between the chest and the abdomen, is weak at the point where the esophagus passes through it into the abdomen. Unusual abdominal pressure, due to pregnancy or to obesity, or a congenital weakness of the diaphragm, may cause a gap to develop in the muscle at this point. Symptoms include burping, hiccups, and heartburn, particularly when bending forward or lying down. The pain may resemble angina pectoris.

TREATMENT. Lose weight if obese. Sleep propped up on several pillows. Eat a small evening meal and use antacid drugs. Occasionally an operation may be necessary to close the gap in the diaphragm muscle.

Hiccups. Repeated involuntary spasms of the diaphragm muscle accompanied by a closure of the vocal cords. Each spasm causes a sharp inhalation of breath and a characteristic sound. They seldom have a serious origin and are usually caused by eating too fast or by sparkling drinks. Hiccups seldom last longer than an hour. Rarely, hiccups may be prolonged due to serious disease, such as kidney failure or diaphragmatic irritation from an infection.

TREATMENT. See FIRST AID: Hiccups, p.37.

Hunchback. This may be a severe form of bent or curved back or it may be due to tuberculosis of the spine in childhood, which causes the collapse of one or two vertebrae leading to the deformity.

TREATMENT. To be successful, treatment must begin as soon as the disorder starts to develop.

Hypochondria. An abnormal anxiety about one's health. It may involve imagined illness accompanied by actual pain, and may be associated with anxiety or depression. It may also indicate personal insecurity that requires repeated reassurance from the authority of a doctor.

Hysteria. A mental state in which the conscious mind is unaware of the real reason for certain thoughts or actions. Hysteria is also regarded as a violent expression of emotion, usually tearful, but this is not the psychiatric use of the term and such emotional outbursts are rarely pathological. In the psychiatric sense, the hysterical patient is genuinely unaware that the pain or illness is imaginary even though there is no medical evidence to support the complaint.

I

Immunization. Immunization provides protection against disease. The more common diseases against which protection may be obtained are listed below, together with recommendations for immunization. Each of the diseases listed is also described in a separate article in the A–Z.

Cholera. Two injections, one to four weeks apart, are required before travelling to places where cholera is endemic. An international certificate takes effect six days after the first injection and lasts for six months. A booster injection may be given within that time. Immunization gives only moderate protection.

Diphtheria. An injection is usually given at the same time as tetanus and whooping cough (pertussis) immunization as triple antigen (DTP), at the ages of five, six and 12 months. A booster injection is required at five years.

German measles (rubella). A single subcutaneous injection may be given at the age of one. Alternatively, girls aged about

11 years may be immunized.

Hepatitis. A vaccine against Hepatitis B is now available.

Influenza. Immunization gives about 70% protection for about six months. The specific vaccine varies each year to combat the particular virus prevalent at that time.

Measles. Immunization at the age of 15 months gives 98% protection. The injection may produce mild catarrh, fever and a slight rash about ten days later. It will protect against natural infection if it is given within three days of contact.

Mumps. Immunization is not routinely given but can be useful to protect adults who have not had mumps. It will not protect if the patient is already in quarantine.

Poliomyelitis. An oral vaccine is given at the same time as immunization for diphtheria, tetanus and whooping cough. Boosters are required at the ages of five and ten years.

Rabies. Vaccine can be used for those who are at particular hazard, e.g. vets, or immediately after a person has been bitten by a possibly infected animal.

Tetanus. Immunization is usually given at the same time as diphtheria and whooping cough immunization (triple antigen). A booster is required at the age of five and then repeated every five years or after a dirty wound or cut.

Tuberculosis. This vaccine, also known as the BCG vaccine, can be given to those who have a negative skin test and who have been in contact with tuberculosis. Immunization usually gives life-long protection.

Typhoid. Partial protection is achieved from two injections given two to four weeks apart. A booster is required every two years. The vaccine often causes a feverish reaction and a sore arm for about a day.

Typhus. Two subcutaneous injections are given a week apart. An international certificate may be required.

Whooping cough (pertussis). This is usually given at the same time as diphtheria and tetanus immunization (triple antigen). In rare cases it may cause a severe reaction and this possibility should be discussed with a doctor before starting the injections. It is not advisable for infants who have had *convulsions*, or who have a family history of severe *allergy* or *eczema*.

Yellow fever. Protection lasts about ten years starting ten days after one injection. An international certificate is required by many countries.

Temporary immunization. This can be given with gamma globulin. It will protect against certain diseases, such as viral *hepatitis*, for three or four months, and may be given when individuals are particularly likely to catch the illness or have already been in contact.

Impetigo. A contagious infection occurring around the mouth and nose. It affects children in particular. Symptoms include blisters that form crusts and spread across the face, hands or knees. It is usually more severe in people who suffer from *eczema*.

TREATMENT. Consult a doctor for an appropriate antibiotic ointment. Cleanliness of body, hands and nails is necessary to prevent a recurrence of the disease.

Incontinence. The inability to hold urine because of failure to control the sphincter muscle that closes the opening from the bladder into the urethra. It is a problem of the elderly but may also affect men who suffer from *prostate problems*, and women in whom the bladder is compressed either during *pregnancy* or by a *prolapse of the womb*. Incontinence usually occurs if the bladder is compressed when laughing or coughing. It may also occur during sleep.

Incontinence of feces, as well as urine, is a much more serious problem and may occur in the elderly who are suffering from confusion and *constipation*, as well as those who have neurological problems, such as *strokes*. See also *Bedwetting*.

TREATMENT. Consult a doctor. Treatment will depend on the cause but if incontinence occurs as a result of prostate or gynecological problems an operation may be required.

Indigestion (dyspepsia). This is vague abdominal discomfort often accompanied by *flatulence, nausea, heartburn, hiccups* and sometimes *abdominal pain*. It may be caused by *anxiety*, heavy *smoking* and drinking as well as an incorrect diet. It may also be a symptom of *gall-bladder disease, gastritis,* an *ulcer* or *hiatus hernia.*

TREATMENT. Take regular, light meals and avoid known causes, for example alcohol, *smoking* and aspirin. Antacid drugs may help. A doctor should always be consulted if symptoms persist.

Infectious mononucleosis (glandular fever). A *herpes* virus infection spread by close contact. Symptoms include *malaise, sore throat, fever,* enlarged spleen, swollen lymph glands, and general weakness. Diagnosis is confirmed by blood tests. The onset is often sudden, and the infection usually lasts for two or three weeks. The main complication found in infectious mononucleosis is *jaundice.*

TREATMENT. Treat as a fever with bed rest during the acute stage. A doctor must be consulted, and care is necessary when giving antibiotics as the body may react abnormally in the course of this disease. A gradual return to normal life is necessary because over-activity may cause a relapse.

Influenza ('flu). A virus infection that commonly reaches epidemic proportions. The type of virus varies from time to time so that immunity to the disease is difficult to acquire. The incubation period of the disease is about 48 hours. Symptoms include the acute onset of fever, sometimes with *vomiting*, a temperature of up to 40°C (104°F), *headache, sore throat,* aching muscles, and often a slight *cough.* An attack usually lasts about three to six days. Complications include *bronchitis, pneumonia, sinusitis,* and *otitis media.*

TREATMENT. Treat as for *fever.* Rest, good ventilation and isolation from others are recommended. Consult a doctor if the cough increases or the temperature remains high. See also *Immunization.*

Insomnia. An inability to sleep. Individuals need different amounts of sleep. Adult requirements vary between four and nine hours every night, babies sleep most of the day, and young children require up to 12 hours a night. Many people wake several times at night and, provided they are not beset by worries, fall asleep again. Insomnia is usually caused by *anxiety, depression*, pain, cold, *fever, indigestion*, stimulants (such as coffee), or drugs.

TREATMENT. A warm milk drink late in the evening and reading a book in bed sometimes help. Avoid sleeping pills, if possible, as they may perpetuate the need to take them. If insomnia persists for more than a few nights, or if health is affected, consult a doctor.

Intussusception. A bowel disorder in which the intestine squeezes
its own internal surface as if it were a piece of food. The result
is that part of the intestine is folded upon itself and this causes
an obstruction. It is commonest in babies and young children.
The symptoms include *vomiting* and *colic*, and sometimes
anal bleeding (see *Anal problems*).
TREATMENT. Urgent surgery is required.

Iritis. Inflammation or infection of the coloured area of the eye.
There are many different causes. Iritis is usually accompanied
by some pain, by blurring of vision and by intolerance of light.
TREATMENT. Iritis requires urgent medical attention.

Irritable bowel syndrome (also known as spastic colon and mucous colitis). A recurrent disorder in which there are bouts of
mild *abdominal pain* with *diarrhea* and *constipation* in an
otherwise healthy person. This may be triggered off by *anxiety*
or food *allergy*, but frequently it occurs for no obvious reason.
The diagnosis is usually made by your doctor, after excluding
more serious conditions such as *diverticulitis* and *colitis.*
TREATMENT. Bulk foods, such as bran, and antispasmodic drugs
are used in treatment.

Itching (known medically as pruritus). An intense, unpleasant
sensation in the skin surface. The reasons are not completely
understood. It may be a symptom of *eczema, scabies, nettle
rash* and many skin disorders. It may also occur with generalized conditions such as *kidney* failure and *jaundice*. Itching of
the eyes may be due to mild *conjunctivitis, hay fever* or mild
infection. Itching round the anus may be due to *hemorrhoids*
or pin*worms*. Vulval itching may be a symptom of *diabetes*.
TREATMENT. Antihistamine drugs may help but a diagnosis by
your doctor is needed for appropriate treatment.

J

Jaundice. Diseases that affect the normal excretion of yellow bile
pigment (bilirubin) into the intestine, and so give a yellow
colour to the skin and whites of the eyes, are known as
jaundice. Specific causes include *cirrhosis* of the liver and
forms of *hepatitis*, blockage of the bile duct (see *Gall-bladder
disease*), and the excessive destruction of red blood cells found
in hemolytic *anemia*. Occasionally jaundice can be caused by
other infectious illnesses or by drugs. See *Yellow fever*.

K

Kidney disorders. The body's blood supply is filtered by the two
kidneys to maintain the correct balance of water and salts.
Waste substances, such as urea and uric acid, are excreted with
the excess of salt and water. Symptoms of kidney disease
include *backache, urine* problems, pus or blood in the *urine*,
and *fever*. Kidney disease may be detected by examination of
the blood and urine and by X-rays following the injection of a
dye into the circulation. This test, an intravenous pyelogram,
depends on the dye being detected by the X-rays as it is
excreted through the kidneys.

Congenital abnormalities of the kidneys, such as cysts, double kidneys and double ureters, may all occur and these make
infection or stone formation more likely.
TREATMENT. In all cases a doctor must be consulted, and hos-

pitalization for assessment of the disorder is usually required. See also *Nephritis* and *Pyelonephritis*.

Knock-knee (genu valgum). This is a common deformity, at the age of about three or four years, following *bow-legs*. There is no need to treat it as it will almost always improve naturally. If it is still present when the child is ten years old, surgical treatment may be required.

L

Laryngitis. Acute laryngitis is caused by a *sore throat* that affects the vocal cords. Chronic laryngitis occurs if the vocal cords continue to be used during an acute attack. The inflammation is aggravated by smoking and alcohol.
TREATMENT. Rinse the mouth regularly and gargle with an antiseptic mouth wash. Try to speak as softly and as little as possible. If the symptoms persist, consult a doctor.

Leukemia. Leukemia is cancer of the white blood cells. In most cases the causes are not known. It may develop suddenly or gradually. The symptoms include *sore throat, fever, malaise,* swollen glands and *anemia.*
TREATMENT. The effectiveness of treatment depends on the type of leukemia. Chemotherapy, using cancer-killing drugs, is the standard form of treatment.

Lice (nits, crabs). Small parasites that infest the skin of mammals and birds. They bite to suck blood from the host, and cause *itching* and scratching. The eggs are often laid in the host's hair. Three types affect humans. Head lice (nits) are most often encountered in children. They are not an indication of lack of cleanliness so much as of shared clothes and towels, usually at school. Body lice are more commonly associated with a lack of hygiene. These are the parasites which are usually responsible for the spread of *typhus*, plague, and other infectious illnesses. The third type of louse is the pubic or crab louse which inhabits the hairs of the pubic region and is transmitted by sexual contact. The names of these parasites indicate the region in which they are usually found, but each type may also be encountered elsewhere.
TREATMENT. Insecticide powder, anti-louse shampoos and lotions and careful removal of eggs help to eradicate the parasites. If lice remain, consult a doctor.

Lightening. This usually occurs in the last few weeks of *pregnancy* when the baby's head settles deep into the mother's pelvis. Lightening leaves more room in the mother's abdomen and this gives an associated feeling of comfort. It may be accompanied by the need to *urinate frequently* because of pressure on the bladder.

Liver disease. Many symptoms of mild ill health are wrongly attributed to disorders of the liver. Despite this reputation, the liver is an organ of unusual efficiency and resilience, able to continue normal functions even when substantially diseased. Causes of liver disease include *alcoholism, gall-bladder disease, hepatitis* and some tropical diseases. Symptoms may be no more obvious than a vague *malaise* and loss of appetite, sometimes accompanied by *jaundice* and tenderness in the upper abdomen. *Cirrhosis* of the liver describes fibrous scarring of the internal structure of the liver. This may be caused by poisons such as alcohol or carbon tetrachloride, by nutritional deficiency or by disease.

Lumbago. A term for low *backache* in the lumbar region.

Lymphogranuloma venereum. A viral *venereal disease* causing
H lymph gland swelling and genital ulceration. It is commoner in tropical countries.

M

Malaise (listlessness, fatigue). Vague symptoms associated with most illnesses, particularly if the onset of an illness or disease is gradual. Listlessness is a characteristic symptom of recovery from an illness or an operation, but in some cases is associated with *depression*.
TREATMENT. Continued listlessness, without obvious cause, requires medical examination. If there is a suspected cause, consult a doctor for advice about the best means of treating it.

Malaria. A tropical illness caused by a unicellular organism (plas-
H modium) transmitted by the bite of the Anopheles mosquito. Symptoms include intermittent high *fever*, sometimes with *delirium*, recurring every few days depending on the type of infection. Malignant malaria causes blockage of the blood vessels, coma, *kidney* failure and death. Prolonged, recurrent malaria produces *anemia* and listlessness.
TREATMENT. Antimalarial drugs are required after careful diagnosis and study by a specialist in tropical medicine. Anyone who develops a fever and who has recently been to a malarious area must consult a doctor at once.

Those intending to visit a malarious region can be protected by regular medication with antimalarial drugs. The drugs should be taken throughout the stay and should be continued for a month after leaving the area. Mosquito netting around the bed is also recommended.

Mania. A state of nervous excitement with an abnormally selfish motivation. Over-enthusiasm, extreme talkativeness, lack of normal inhibitions, failure to maintain a consistent course of action, intolerance of others and a supreme feeling of righteousness are typical symptoms. These are often accompanied by great physical activity and an increased sex drive.
TREATMENT. Sedative drugs and skilled psychiatric care are required. Sometimes compulsory hospital treatment is necessary to prevent exhaustion.

Manic-depressive illness. An abnormal mental state characterized by periods of *mania* and severe *depression*. The intensity of the attacks may vary and they are usually separated by periods of relative stability. The illness should not be confused with the normal fluctuations of mood which are a characteristic feature of adolescence.
TREATMENT. The instability of the manic-depressive may be controlled with drugs, but a careful diagnosis by a doctor or psychiatrist is required before any treatment is initiated.

Mastoiditis. An acute or chronic infection of the bone behind the ear, usually caused by the spread of infection from *otitis media*.

TREATMENT. Consult a doctor. Large doses of antibiotics usually cure mastoiditis but occasionally an operation (mastoidectomy) is needed to remove the infected bone.

Masturbation. Most babies sooner or later find pleasure in touching their own genitals. Boys will have erections due to a full bladder as well as from masturbation. Rocking movements that rub the genitals often produce a flushed, almost trance-like state followed by relaxation and sleep. This does no harm. The baby or child should not be reprimanded or punished but, if possible, should be distracted by some more sociable occupation. Most children grow out of this stage when young and return to it at puberty. In rare cases, compulsive masturbation, to the exclusion of normal life, is a sign of insecurity and anxiety. This will require skilled psychiatric help for the child and the family.

Masturbation in adolescence and adult life is not harmful and is a normal release of sexual tension in those for whom sexual intercourse may not be possible. The frequency varies greatly from person to person. See *Sexuality*.

Measles (rubeola). A virus infection, the symptoms of which include *fever* with *catarrh, sore throat* and *conjunctivitis* for three to five days before the onset of a fine, pink-red *rash* that starts behind the ears and spreads over the face and down to the trunk and limbs. The incubation period may be up to two weeks, but is usually about ten days. Measles is infectious from the onset of fever until five days after the rash appears. For one or two days before the rash, tiny red spots with white centres (Koplik's spots) may be noticed inside the cheeks or on the palate. A dry, unproductive *cough*, a *headache* and profound *malaise* are present throughout the illness. Complications include *bronchitis, otitis media, sinusitis*, and, rarely, *encephalitis*.

TREATMENT. Treat as a *fever*. The patient should be isolated in a well-ventilated room, with the curtains drawn if the eyes are painful. Complications will require a doctor's diagnosis and treatment with antibiotics. Severe cases, and those with *encephalitis*, need hospital treatment.

Quarantine: Two weeks after last contact with the disease. See also *Immunization*.

Melanoma. A dark, pigmented lesion on the skin. It may become malignant, so any change in size or colour of a skin lesion must be shown to a doctor. Malignant melanomas are very rare in children but commoner, as with all forms of skin *cancer*, in those who have spent much of their lives in strong sunlight. It is more common in lesions on the legs, under the nails and in the pigmented area at the back of the eye, and it is also seen more frequently in women than men.

TREATMENT. Immediate surgery is required, followed, if necessary, by cytotoxic drugs.

Ménière's disease. A disease caused by an intermittent increase of fluid pressure in the inner ear. It usually occurs in people over the age of about 40. In one case out of four both ears become involved. The cause is not known. Symptoms include intermittent attacks of giddiness, buzzing in the ear, *nausea, vomiting*, and gradually increasing *deafness* over a number of years. Each attack lasts from minutes to hours but the buzzing can continue all the time and lead to *depression*.

TREATMENT. It may help to lie down and take antinausea medication. In long-term treatment a variety of drugs are used, and sometimes an operation can cure the disease.

Meningitis. An inflammation of the membranes surrounding the brain and spinal cord, caused by viral or bacterial infections. **H** Symptoms include a severe *headache, fever,* intolerance of light, stiff neck, and *vomiting.* Meningitis may damage the brain and nervous system, and may prove fatal.

TREATMENT. Urgent admission to a hospital for investigation and treatment with antibiotics is vital. The patient should be isolated. Darkness and quiet are essential as excitement may cause the patient to have *convulsions.* See also *Encephalitis.*

Menopause. This usually occurs between the ages of 45 and 55 and signifies the end of menstruation. The menopause is also known as the female climacteric. It may be preceded by several months of irregular menstruation and it is associated with other symptoms caused by the gradual hormonal changes that occur at this age. *Depression,* loss of sexual interest, flushes, palpitations or tension may also occur.

TREATMENT. Many women do not have any symptoms that worry or concern them and do not need treatment. Others may find the symptoms distressing and a doctor can help with various treatments, including hormone replacement therapy. Any *vaginal bleeding* that occurs more than six months after the last period may indicate a serious disorder, such as *cancer,* and a doctor must be consulted.

Menstrual disorders. Irregular bleeding, bleeding that occurs too frequently or heavily (see *Vaginal bleeding*), or the absence of periods (amenorrhea) is usually due to hormonal disorders. Amenorrhea may be due to *pregnancy,* early *menopause, anorexia nervosa, anxiety,* or any severe or prolonged illness. It may also occur after oral *contraception* has been stopped.

TREATMENT. Discuss the symptoms with a doctor. If menstruation has stopped, have a *pregnancy test* to exclude early *pregnancy.* If necessary, hormonal treatment or a *D and C* operation may be required. Amenorrhea is only rarely a symptom of a more serious complaint and usually it is best to wait until menstruation restarts naturally.

Migraine. Severe recurring *headaches* often accompanied by *nausea* and disturbed vision. They are frequently one-sided. The causes are not known. Often the first signs of a migraine attack are visual disorders such as a narrowed field of vision or flashing lights in front of the eyes. These effects are usually followed by a severe one-sided headache with a dislike of light and noise. In children recurrent attacks of *vomiting* may be the prelude to the development of typical migraine headaches as they grow older.

TREATMENT. Effervescent aspirin taken as soon as possible at the start of an attack is the most effective treatment. Lie down in a quiet place. Consult a doctor or an organization that specializes in the study of migraine for advice.

Miscarriage. A lay term for *abortion,* the loss of a baby before the **H** 28th week of *pregnancy,* usually in the first three months. At least 10% of all pregnancies end in a miscarriage. Most are due to an abnormality in the fetus, but some are due to hormonal imbalance and a few to weakness in the neck of the womb, illness or severe trauma. The principal symptom is *vaginal bleeding* during pregnancy. This is abnormal and must be regarded as a sign of a threatened miscarriage. If there is pain and loss of tissue, miscarriage is inevitable.

TREATMENT. If there is heavy bleeding, possibly accompanied by *backache* and cramp-like pain, lie down on a plastic sheet covered with towelling and have an extra towel available to staunch further bleeding. Inform a doctor at once. If heavy bleeding continues the doctor will arrange urgent admission to a hospital. The doctor should also be consulted if there is light bleeding without pain. Remain in bed until no further bleeding has occurred for at least 24 hours. Initial bleeding is bright red but this will become brown, indicating old blood, as it settles. See also FIRST AID: Miscarriage, p.38.

Moniliasis (candidiasis, thrush). A fungal infection that most commonly affects the vagina although it can develop in other warm, moist areas of the body, e.g. under the breasts or in the groin. In babies the mouth may be affected, leaving a typically white, speckly appearance of "thrush." It causes soreness and discomfort, producing pain on feeding in babies, and a *vaginal discharge* in women. Moniliasis can be sexually transmitted; the woman may not notice any symptoms, but the man carries the infection.

TREATMENT. Consult a doctor for appropriate antifungal treatment. If a woman is being treated for infection her sexual partner may also be given treatment to prevent reinfection.

Morning sickness. This affects about 50% of women during early *pregnancy*. It is seldom severe but may be aggravated by *anxiety* or travelling.

TREATMENT. Small meals eaten at frequent intervals, and a drink of milk and a biscuit before moving in the morning, prevent an excess of gastric secretions. Certain drugs taken in early pregnancy may harm a fetus and a doctor must be consulted before antinausea drugs are used.

Multiple sclerosis. A chronic disease of the nervous system. It develops over many years during which time increasingly severe attacks alternate with apparent recovery. Symptoms include double vision, weakness, local numbness, dizziness, difficulty in speaking, increasing *paralysis* and *blindness*. The cause of the disease is not known, although it rarely starts in people more than 40 years old.

TREATMENT. Corticosteroid drugs may ease individual attacks. Practical advice may be obtained from charitable associations that exist to help victims of multiple sclerosis and to promote research.

Mumps. A virus infection that causes inflammation and swelling ☎ of the parotid and other salivary glands in the mouth and throat. Symptoms develop gradually with *headache*, slight *fever* and pain behind the ears leading to marked swelling of the parotid glands beneath the angle of the jaw. The swelling usually lasts for about a week. The most serious complications are inflammation of the testicles in adult males and the breasts and ovaries in women, which may cause sterility. Occasionally mumps may also cause *deafness*.

TREATMENT. Treat as a *fever*, with bed rest, plenty of fluids, and a diet that does not require chewing. Cold compresses may help to control swelling of the testicles. Immunization is also possible.

Quarantine: 28 days from last contact with the disease. See also *Immunization*.

N

Nausea. An unpleasant sensation of being about to vomit, often associated with *abdominal* discomfort, which may actually lead to *vomiting*. It may be caused by any disturbance or infection of the digestive system (*gastritis*), by disturbance or disease of the organ of balance in the ear, as in *travel sickness*, by virus infections of the ear, by *migraine*, or as a side-effect of some drugs. Nausea may also be associated with *pregnancy (morning sickness)* or use of the pill (see *Contraception*).
TREATMENT. This must be directed at the cause, but sips of water, anti-indigestion medicines and antinausea drugs may help. A few long deep breaths may also alleviate the symptoms of acute nausea. Lie down if possible.

Nearsightedness (myopia). Difficulty in seeing distant objects indicates myopia. Nearsightedness is considered to be an inherited tendency. It is corrected by wearing glasses.

Nephritis. An inflammation of the kidney, commonly due to streptococcal infection; may be associated with *scarlet fever*. Symptoms include *backache*, swollen *eyelids* and ankles, rapid pulse, *fever, vomiting*, and blood in the *urine*. In its acute form the illness may last 2–3 weeks during which the patient should be in a hospital. If the disease becomes chronic *kidney* failure may ultimately occur.
TREATMENT. A doctor must be consulted and hospitalization is often required. Absolute bed rest is essential, with a diet that is low in protein and salt. Antibiotics are given to kill the streptococcal infection. See also *Rheumatic fever* and *Strep throat*.

Nettle rash (urticaria). A transient eruption of pale, itching swellings. It may be caused by jellyfish or nettle stings, insect bites, a mild *allergy* to certain foods or drugs, or it may be a reaction to emotions such as *anxiety* and *depression*.
TREATMENT. A cold compress, a soothing lotion, and antihistamine drugs often relieve the symptoms. See also FIRST AID: Insect bites and stings, p.37.

Neurosis. A common and usually minor type of mental disorder experienced in some form or other by most people. It may be caused by some *anxiety* or experience (trauma), or by unresolved conflicts. Symptoms of neurosis may resemble fatigue, nervousness, *depression*, fear, *obsession* or *hysteria*.

Night sweats. These are common in healthy children who have been active all day and whose body temperature drops suddenly when asleep. A night sweat is normal even if it is so severe that the child's night-clothes are soaked. Night sweats may also occur in adults who use too many bedclothes or keep an electric blanket on at night. They may also occur in any illness that is associated with *fever*. If they occur irregularly over a long period, consult a doctor.

Night terrors. Babies may wake terrified and screaming during the night. If old enough, a child may be able to describe a nightmare but often it is unable to do so. Night terrors may occur frequently for a period of time and then cease. At some time or another they are common in most young children. They may be due to an active imagination or to more deep-seated anxiety and insecurity.

TREATMENT. Reassurance and cuddling from a parent until the child is sleepy again is the only immediate treatment. It is rarely necessary to consult a doctor unless night terrors recur very frequently.

Nonspecific urethritis (NSU). This is inflammation of the urethra not due to any specific infection. NSU is transmitted through sexual intercourse but is caused by non-gonorrheal organisms. Symptoms resemble those of *gonorrhea*. In men they include painful urination and discharge from the *penis*. In women symptoms include a red and swollen vulva and a *vaginal discharge*.

TREATMENT. Consult a doctor. The discharge must be examined so that the cause of infection can be identified. Treatment with antibiotics may be required.

Nosebleed (epistaxis). Hemorrhage from the nose may be caused by *colds, catarrh*, blowing the nose too hard, injury, foreign bodies in the nasal passage or changes in atmospheric pressure. It may also be associated with *arteriosclerosis*, violent exertion, bleeding disorders or with the hormonal changes of puberty and menstruation.

TREATMENT. See FIRST AID: Nosebleed, p.39.

O

Obesity. The condition of being excessively overweight as a result of an imbalance between food intake and energy output. It may be due to *thyroid problems* or other endocrine disorders but it is usually caused by the habit of overeating which may be aggravated by *depression* and *anxiety*. It causes *breathlessness* and may predispose the sufferer to skin problems, *heart* disease, *arthritis*, and *diabetes*.

TREATMENT. Consult your doctor for suitable dietary recommendations. Appetite-depressant drugs may be prescribed and hormone disorders treated if necessary.

Obsession. A common form of *neurosis* characterized by a recurring idea that compels the individual to do something to relieve an exaggerated sense of *anxiety*. It is most likely to occur in a minor form. Severe forms of obsession may cause great inconvenience, and may develop to the point where they dominate the waking hours of the patient's life.

Osteoporosis. A bone disorder in which both calcium and bone fabric are lost – unlike *rickets* and osteomalacia in adults, when only calcium is lost due to lack of Vitamin D. It occurs in people over 50, more frequently in women, and usually there are no symptoms. The spine becomes shorter, causing a *bent back*, and sometimes pressure on spinal nerves causes pain. *Fractures* occur more easily if the person falls. The condition is difficult to treat as it is part of aging. Some forms of hormone therapy may help.

Otitis externa. An infection of the outer tube of the ear. It may be caused by a form of *eczema*, by swimming, particularly in hot climates, by scratching the ears with the finger nails, and occasionally by excess *wax*. Symptoms include *itching*, slight *ear discharging, earache, deafness*, or *fever*.

TREATMENT. Keep water out and do not scratch the ear. Consult a doctor for the appropriate treatment with antibiotic ear drops. Clean excess wax from the ears.

Otitis media. An infection of the middle ear. It is usually associated with a *cold* and *catarrh* blocking the Eustachian tube, with ☎ acute *tonsillitis*, or with flying or diving while suffering from catarrh. Symptoms include *earache, deafness, fever*, and *ear discharging* if the eardrum bursts.

TREATMENT. Immediate treatment is necessary, using nose drops, antihistamines and pain-killing drugs followed by antibiotics from a doctor. Do not use ear drops. Inadequate treatment may lead to *mastoiditis* or *deafness*.

P

Paleness (pallor). Paleness indicates a reduced blood supply to the skin and may be a sign of cold, fatigue, recent illness, shock, or *anemia*. If it persists, a doctor should be consulted.

Palpitations. The normal pulse rate in an adult at rest is about 70 or 80 beats a minute. Rapid regular beats (tachycardia) occur after exercise. An increased pulse rate can also be detected because of *anxiety, smoking*, an overactive *thyroid*, or some forms of *heart* disease. Slow, regular beats (bradycardia) are found in the trained athlete at rest. Bradycardia is also characteristic of an underactive *thyroid*. Missed beats (ventricular extrasystoles) may occasionally occur in the normal heart at rest. They are also caused by *smoking* and they may be a sign of *heart* disease. Irregular rapid beats (atrial fibrillation) and other irregularities are usually symptoms of *heart* disease. Any uncertainties about the condition of the heart should be discussed with a doctor at the earliest available opportunity. A thorough examination may be necessary to exclude the possibility of heart disease.

Paralysis. Loss of strength in a muscle or group of muscles. It is indicated by obvious disability and also by impairment of ☎ specific functions such as blinking, speech, urination or use of a limb. Paralysis is usually due to damage to the nervous system caused by a disease such as *polyneuritis* or *poliomyelitis*, by a *stroke* or by an injury. It may also be psychological in origin (see *Hysteria*), and if no other symptoms appear this possibility should be investigated.

TREATMENT. The cause must be determined, usually by hospital investigation. During recovery it is important to keep the muscles active, and treatment and advice from a physiotherapist are necessary.

Paranoia. A severe mental disorder in which delusions of persecution affect a person's way of life and reactions to outside situations. The characteristics of a paranoiac include suspicion, self-consciousness, and logical explanations of the delusions which support an increasing web of dislikes and fears. Paranoia may be dangerous because the patient believes that the persecution is real, and so may act violently as a result of this delusion.

TREATMENT. Psychiatric therapy is necessary to rehabilitate mild cases. Severe cases require permanent care.

Parkinson's disease. A nervous disease characterized by trembling and muscular weakness. It usually develops gradually from a slight trembling of the hands over several years to generalized muscular debility. The disease, most common in the elderly, does not affect intelligence.

TREATMENT. Anti-Parkinsonian drugs, particularly Levodopa, are usually effective but severe cases may need brain surgery. Chest and respiratory disorders must be treated at once to prevent further complications. See *Encephalitis*.

Penis, discharge from. This is always a sign of infection. It may be
H caused by any venereal disease, but most commonly it is due to *nonspecific urethritis*.

TREATMENT. Both patient and sexual partner must consult a doctor and abstain from sexual intercourse until cured. See *Gonorrhea* and *Venereal diseases*.

Periods (menstruation). The onset (menarche) of periods is usually between the ages of ten and 14. They cease at the *menopause*, between the ages of 45 and 55. At first they may be irregular, and vary in length and amount of bleeding. After two or three years most girls settle into a regular rhythm. The first day of bleeding is the first day of the menstrual cycle, the period of bleeding lasts four to six days and the next cycle begins with the onset of the next period. Cycles generally last between 26 and 30 days. Some women may have a longer (e.g. six-week) or a shorter (e.g. three-week) cycle.

Ovulation, the production of the egg, usually occurs in the middle of the cycle, 14 days before menstruation begins. Periods may occur without ovulation and it is also possible to ovulate without having had a period for some time.

When the periods first start, external sanitary towels are usually found to be easiest to use. A girl should be instructed in their use and her mother should advise her before the event as the first period can be frightening if it occurs unexpectedly. When periods are regular, and the girl is physically larger, internal tampons are frequently used. The use of internal tampons requires a little practice and care. After a period, douching with warm water or a warm weak solution of bicarbonate of soda is unlikely to do harm but stronger chemicals should not be used. Reasonable external washing and careful drying are all that are required.

Periods, painful (dysmenorrhea). In older women pain may be due to *salpingitis*, to an inflammation of the uterus, or it may be associated with *premenstrual tension* and last throughout the period. Between the ages of 15 and 25 cramping pain in the lower abdomen, sometimes with *backache* and pain down either side of the thighs, may start 24 hours before, and last for 24 to 48 hours after, the start of the period.

TREATMENT. A doctor should be consulted. Treatment should be started before the pain begins, if possible, and should continue throughout the period. Do not wait for the pain to return or become severe. Many women are helped by simple pain-killing drugs taken every four hours. The contraceptive pill may have a beneficial side-effect in stopping painful periods. In some cases, a *D and C* operation may be required.

Peritonitis. An infection of the membrane that lines the abdomen
H and surrounds the abdominal organs. Peritonitis may be caused by an infection or rupture of an abdominal structure.

This may occur in *appendicitis, salpingitis, diverticulitis,* or as a result of a burst peptic *ulcer.* Symptoms include severe *abdominal pain, fever,* and often *vomiting.*

TREATMENT. Immediate admission to a hospital is required for an operation to drain the infection, followed by skilled nursing care and antibiotic treatment.

Phlebitis. The inflammation of a vein, usually in the leg. It occurs most commonly as a result of childbirth, *varicose veins,* or an operation. The skin above the vein is tender and may be discoloured. Swelling of the leg may also occur. The inflammation may lead to the formation of a blood clot (thrombophlebitis). See *Thrombosis.*

TREATMENT. The leg should be firmly bandaged and the patient should be encouraged to move. Pain-killing and anti-inflammatory drugs may be prescribed. A hot compress placed on the inflamed area may help temporarily. Movement maintains the circulation in the affected limb.

Pleurisy. An infection of the pleural membrane that lines the chest cavity and surrounds the lungs. Inflammation causes extreme pain in the chest when breathing, coughing or moving. Pleurisy may be caused by *pneumonia, cancer,* an *embolus* or an infection from a wound.

TREATMENT. Consult a doctor immediately so that the correct treatment can be given. Sit propped up in bed with a hot pad over the painful side. Antibiotics will probably be required, and a sedative cough mixture and pain-killing drugs may also be prescribed. See also CHART OF WHAT TO DO: Chest pain, p.95.

Pneumoconiosis. A general term for lung disorders due to inhalation of dust. Coal, iron and many dusts are apparently harmless, but rock dust, causing silicosis, produces *emphysema* and *bronchitis.* Asbestos, causing asbestosis, may lead to lung *cancer* as well. Dusts from plants and fibres, e.g. cotton, may produce *asthma.*

Pneumonia. A serious infection of lung tissue. It occurs most commonly as bronchopneumonia which may develop as an extension of *bronchitis.* Lobar pneumonia, an infection of an anatomical segment of the lungs, may also occur. Pneumonia is caused by a variety of bacteria or viruses. The symptoms include *cough, fever* and *pleurisy.* These may develop suddenly or gradually following a *cold* or *bronchitis.*

TREATMENT. Appropriate antibiotics are necessary, and breathing exercises, steam inhalations, pain-killing drugs and cough mixtures also help. It is essential to stop *smoking.* Pneumonia is particularly serious in the elderly and in those suffering from any other serious illness.

Poker back. This is due to rigidity of the lower spine caused by the rheumatic condition, ankylosing *spondylitis.* See also *Bent or curved back.*

Poliomyelitis. An infection of the spinal cord caused by the water-borne polio virus. The symptoms of the minor form of polio include mild *fever, headache,* stiff neck and muscle ache, and last for two or three days. In the major form of polio, which is less common, these symptoms are followed by the rapid onset of high *fever,* muscle pains, intolerance of light, and severe *headache.* The final stage is the weakness or *paralysis* of some muscles which may limit breathing and sometimes cause death. Only about 10% of those infected with poliomyelitis develop the major form of the illness and not all of these are left paralysed. The symptoms appear about two or three weeks after the victim has caught the disease and it remains infectious for a further three weeks.

TREATMENT. Isolation in a hospital with complete rest. Pain-killing drugs and artificial respiration may be needed. *Immunization* of children is strongly advised and anyone who has been in contact with the disease should be revaccinated.

Polyneuritis. An inflammation of more than one nerve. Symptoms include numbness, tingling, muscle pain, double vision, weakness and *paralysis*, and may be due to poisoning by lead, insecticides or other chemicals; to *diabetes, vitamin B* deficiency, or infections such as *diphtheria* or *mumps*; or to *cancer*, often cancer of the lung.

TREATMENT. The cause must be determined and, if the symptoms are severe, treated in a hospital. Physiotherapy and vitamin B supplements may assist recovery.

Polyp. A growth occurring anywhere of the mucous membranes lining the inside of the body, commonly in the nose, often associated with *hay fever* and *catarrh*, or in the large intestine where they may become cancerous. If they cause problems, such as nasal or intestinal obstruction, they must be removed.

Pregnancy. Pregnancy lasts for about 280 days from the moment of conception (fertilization of the ovum by the sperm) in the Fallopian tube until the end of the second stage of labour (*childbirth*) when the baby is born. The expected day of delivery (EDD) is calculated as nine months and seven days after the first day of the last period. During the first three months indications of pregnancy include swollen and tender breasts (see *Breast problems*), *morning sickness*, and minimal weight gain. In the second three months, *quickening* occurs with gradual weight gain and evidence of increasing abdominal growth. In the final three months there is a faster increase in weight and size before *lightening* and labour occur.

Antenatal care of pregnant women should include a blood test and regular examination by an obstetrician of urine, blood pressure and weight to protect against toxemia of pregnancy, rhesus factor incompatibility, *anemia*, and *venereal disease*. Abdominal examination should be conducted to ensure that the baby is growing correctly. An obstetrician will also give advice about diet (and extra vitamins and iron that may be required), general exercise, rest, special exercises to help in labour, and postnatal care of the baby.

Pregnancy test. A test for pregnancy can be performed on urine that has been collected in a clean bottle. The bottle must not contain any traces of detergents, soap or other chemicals. A pharmacist can perform the test or, with some preparations, the test can be done at home, but it will not be effective until at least ten days after the missed period. Occasionally the result may remain negative, despite repeated tests, even when the woman is pregnant, but it is extremely rare for the result to be positive when pregnancy has not occurred.

Premenstrual tension. This may occur during the week preceding a period, particularly as a woman gets older. It is usually associated with fluid retention, which gives a feeling of abdominal distension. Symptoms include breast tenderness (see *Breast problems*), weight gain, *headaches*, and occasionally spots on the face and shoulders. Premenstrual tension may also lead to *anxiety* and *depression*.

TREATMENT. Discussion with a doctor may give reassurance that this is a physical and not a psychological illness. Diuretics (fluid-removing drugs) will often help if they are taken for at least a week before the period is due.

Prolapse. An abnormal downward displacement of part of the body – either the womb or the rectum.

☎ **Prolapse of the rectum.** A relatively rare occurrence in which the mucosal lining of the rectum separates from the muscle wall and hangs out through the anus. This may occur spontaneously in infants. It may also be caused by *hemorrhoids* or recurrent *constipation*. It appears as a bulge of soft, red tissue hanging out of the anus.

TREATMENT. In infants it is self-curing. In adults the excess mucosa may be cut off in an operation and the edges joined together, or the patient may be given special injections which produce scarring and thereby cause the mucosa to adhere to the muscle wall. In certain cases a wire ring may be used to narrow the anal opening.

Prolapse of the womb (uterus). This is caused by a weakening of the muscles and ligaments that hold the womb in its normal position. A prolapsed uterus falls into the vagina pulling the bladder and, to a lesser extent, the bowel with it. The uterine ligaments may have been overstretched in *childbirth* or weakened after the *menopause*. The indications of a prolapse are not always obvious but there may be a feeling of pressure, as if something has fallen. Involuntary urination when coughing, laughing or lifting something, *backache* and *depression* may also be associated with a prolapse.

TREATMENT. An operation to tighten the ligaments is usual but in the elderly a plastic ring can be put in the upper end of the vagina to hold the uterus in place.

Prostate problems. The prostate gland is found in men underneath the bladder. As the urethra passes through the gland from the bladder to the penis, it is joined by the two spermatic cords from the testes.

Prostatic enlargement occurs as men get older, and is fairly common over the age of 60. The enlargement distorts the bladder and the urethra. Symptoms of prostatic enlargement include frequent or difficult *urination*, together with hesitant starting and dribbling after finishing. Sometimes an urgent need to urinate is followed by an inability to do so. Slight *incontinence*, sometimes complete *urine retention*, and occasionally blood in the *urine* may also occur. An infection of the prostate (prostatitis) may occur at any age and may be a complication of venereal diseases such as *gonorrhea*. The symptoms resemble those of prostatic enlargement.

TREATMENT. Consult a doctor, as increasingly severe symptoms indicate that an operation is required. This is usually performed through the penis but may sometimes be performed through the abdomen. If *cancer* is found, drug treatment is often effective. Infections of the prostate are usually treated with antibiotics. See also FIRST AID: Urine, unable to pass, p.44.

Psoriasis. A skin disease, characterized by patches of mildly irri-

tated, red, scaling skin. The cause of psoriasis is not known. The symptoms may not appear until adulthood, and they may vary greatly in severity, sometimes disappearing for long periods. They are likely to be aggravated by emotional stress.
TREATMENT. Various skin preparations may help to reduce scaling. Ultraviolet light is beneficial and the use of various strong, cell-killing (cytotoxic) drugs may help severe cases.

Psychosis. An abnormal mental state produced by *alcoholism, schizophrenia, drug abuse* or an underlying illness. Psychosis is indicated by major disorders of personality, often associated with delusions, hallucinations and abnormal behaviour.
TREATMENT. Hospitalization is usually required.

Puberty. Puberty is the stage of growth during which the secondary sexual characteristics develop. A girl's breasts develop and her body acquires the shape of a young woman. A boy's voice deepens and hair starts to grow on his face, arms, legs and chest and in the pubic region. Menstruation (*periods*) and sperm formation start at about the same stage of development so that from this time reproduction is possible. Puberty is associated with the psychological changes of adolescence. These affect not only *sexuality* but also the adolescent's relationships with parents and other adults.

Pyelonephritis. Inflammation of the pelvis of the *kidney*. It may be caused by *pregnancy, cystitis, tuberculosis,* a congenital abnormality or an obstruction to the urine flow. Symptoms include *fever,* chill, frequent and painful *urination, backache* and *vomiting.*
TREATMENT. Antibiotic therapy, pain-killing drugs and bed rest are necessary for recovery. If the infection is not completely cleared it may cause chronic pyelitis and gradual kidney damage leading to kidney failure.

Q

Quickening. The first time a pregnant woman feels her baby move is known as "quickening." It is usually a slight fluttering sensation and is normally felt between the 16th and 20th weeks of pregnancy.

R

Rabies (hydrophobia). A disease caused by a virus transmitted in the saliva of an infected warm-blooded animal, usually by a bite. The animals most commonly responsible for transmitting rabies are dogs, foxes and bats. The incubation period is usually about five weeks, but the symptoms may appear as early as a week or as long as a year after the bite. Symptoms include extreme mental excitement, severe muscle spasms, especially of the throat when drinking, and ultimately respiratory paralysis and death.
TREATMENT. Antirabies vaccine must be given as soon as possible after being bitten by an infected animal. There is no effective treatment of the disease once the symptoms appear. Any animal that appears unusually aggressive should be considered a potential carrier of rabies and should be examined for the disease. Vaccination of an animal may protect it from the disease but immunity is not guaranteed and a quarantine period of six months is also required. See also *Immunization.*

Rash. A pink or red, often *itching*, inflammation of the skin. It is usually a sign of an *allergic* reaction, in which case it is of short duration. It may also be a symptom of certain infectious illnesses, such as *measles* and *chickenpox*, or of a skin infection, and it may be associated with *anxiety*.
TREATMENT. It is important to treat the allergy or disease that causes the rash. Cooling the inflamed area and applying a soothing lotion may give temporary relief.

Raynaud's phenomenon. An intermittent spasm of the small arteries in the fingers and toes, associated with cold. These turn white and numb and then, as they are recovering, become red and painful. The skin may ulcerate.
TREATMENT. Drugs that dilate the blood vessels are used. See also *Chilblain*.

Rheumatic fever. An allergic reaction, related to acute *nephritis* and *scarlet fever*, that affects the heart and joints of children. It is caused by a streptococcal infection. Symptoms include a *sore throat* followed about two weeks later by *fever*, with intermittent painful swelling of the joints. Sometimes there is a blotchy *rash*. All layers of the heart, including the valves, are likely to be involved. The disease lasts many weeks, and the damage to the heart may be permanent.
TREATMENT. Bed rest with large doses of aspirin and nursing care of the joints are required for the duration of the illness. Antibiotics may be required for several years. The patient needs thorough medical assessment.

Rheumatism. A general term used to describe persistent aches in the muscles and joints due to inflammation or other disorders of connective tissue, and frequently associated with cold and damp weather. It is not recognized as a specific disease but may be a symptom of many.
TREATMENT. The disorder that causes the symptoms of rheumatism should be diagnosed and treated. The symptoms may be alleviated by warmth and by drugs such as aspirin.

Rickets (rachitis). A disease, caused by *vitamin D* deficiency, that causes softening and subsequently deformity of the bones, particularly in children. The most obvious deformities are distorted spine, *knock-knees*, *bow-legs*, and pigeon chest. A deficiency of vitamin D in adults will cause calcium to be lost from the bones, leading to osteomalacia.
TREATMENT. As a deficiency disease, rickets can be prevented by sunshine and a balanced diet that provides an adequate intake of vitamin D.

Rodent ulcer (basal cell carcinoma). A malignant ulcer on the skin that does not spread to distant parts. It starts as a small, pearly nodule, usually on the face, and later ulcerates.
TREATMENT. In the early stages it is easily cured by specialist treatment.

Rupture (hernia). Describes not only the breaking or tearing of tissue (as in a ruptured appendix in *appendicitis*) but also a hernia which is due to weakness in the muscles covering part of the abdomen. This weakness allows internal structures to push through the muscle wall. A hernia may occur in the groin (inguinal and femoral hernia), at the umbilicus (umbilical hernia), and occasionally elsewhere, e.g. at the site of a scar or through the diaphragm (see *Hiatus hernia*).

TREATMENT. An operation is the only effective cure for a hernia, but a truss may be helpful as a temporary measure. See also FIRST AID: Hernia, p.37

S

Salpingitis. An inflammation of the ducts (Fallopian tubes) from the ovaries to the uterus. The infecting organisms usually spread from the neck of the womb (cervix) through the womb itself to the Fallopian tubes. The causes include infections of the vagina (*vaginitis*) or the cervix, *venereal disease*, or infection following an *abortion* or *miscarriage*. The symptoms may be acute, with *fever, abdominal pain* and *vaginal discharge*, or chronic, with dull, lower *abdominal pain*.

TREATMENT. A doctor must be consulted. Acute cases require admission to a hospital where the disease is treated with antibiotics and sometimes an operation to drain an abscess. Chronic salpingitis also needs a long course of antibiotics. Complications of salpingitis may be serious and can include *peritonitis* and sterility.

Scabies. A contagious skin infection transmitted by mites. It is spread by close body contact and is easily passed from one member of a family to another. The mite burrows into the skin, usually in the hand or wrist, pubic area, elbows or buttocks. After about a month a red *rash* appears in the infected area as an *allergic* reaction. People who are subsequently reinfected develop the rash within a few hours because the allergy is already present.

TREATMENT. After a bath, dry carefully and paint the whole body, from neck downwards, with an antiscabies preparation. Repeat on the two following days. Change bed linen and clothing and wash the used fabrics with great care.

Scarlet fever (scarlatina). A contagious infection due to streptococcus bacteria that causes a characteristic scarlet rash. The symptoms develop from one to six days after contact and include *sore throat, fever*, rapid pulse, *rash* and inflamed tongue. Peeling skin and thinning hair may also occur.

TREATMENT. Penicillin should be given for at least ten days, following a doctor's advice. The patient should be isolated and kept in bed and the symptoms treated as a *fever*. Antibiotic treatment is necessary to prevent complications such as *rheumatic fever* or *nephritis*.

Quarantine: Until throat swabs are negative.

Scars. Inelastic tissue formed as part of the normal healing process of cut or damaged skin. Keloid scars are thicker than normal because too much fibrous tissue has been produced. These occur after burns, in particular, and in some people who are particularly susceptible. Contraction of large scars may prevent full movement of a joint and such scars often distort the tissues of the face. An irregular, thick, contracted scar may be made less unsightly by plastic surgery.

Schizophrenia. A mental disorder affecting emotion and thought and, ultimately, behaviour. *Psychosis* and *paranoia* are common symptoms. The causes of the disorder are not known, but it has been attributed to various influences, including hereditary factors, chemical imbalance in the brain, upbringing, emotional stress, and *drug abuse.*

TREATMENT. Initially, specialized psychiatric care is required to give the patient confidence in a shared, rather than an isolated, sense of reality. If this is not successful the patient may need compulsory hospital treatment and the use of antipsychotic and tranquillizing drugs. Continued psychiatric care is usually required to prevent relapse.

Sciatica. Pressure on part of the sciatic nerve, which runs from the lower spine down the back of the thigh and leg to the foot, causes *backache*, pain and, sometimes, numbness in the parts of the leg supplied by the nerve. Sciatica is usually caused by *arthritis* of the spine or a *slipped disc.*

TREATMENT. A definite diagnosis must be made by a doctor, if necessary with the aid of X-rays and blood tests. The doctor may prescribe pain-killing and antirheumatic drugs. Physiotherapy can teach correct bending with a straight back and bent knees and can strengthen back muscles.

Sex problems:

Physical. The inability to take part in sexual activities because of a physical difficulty. The problem may be one of ignorance or anxiety about the physical techniques of sexual intercourse, in which case simple explanations given by a doctor are all that are required. If intercourse is painful it may be due to a disorder of the vagina (*vaginitis*) or to some other female problem, or it may be caused by an inflammation of the end of the *penis.* In either case, consult a doctor. The problem may also be one of physical disability. *Paralysis*, a nerve disorder such as *sciatica*, *arthritis*, or illnesses such as *diabetes* may lead to sexual problems, any of which should be discussed with a doctor.

Psychological. Almost all aspects of *sexuality* are affected by a person's mentality, adolescent experience and present state of mind. *Depression* produces a lack of sexual drive and reduces the frequency of intercourse. This requires sympathy and understanding from the healthy partner, and treatment of the cause of depression. Sexual frustration may occur if there is no normal sexual relief, and can lead to *depression*, *anxiety* and irritability. In institutions containing people of only one sex, frustration may lead to *masturbation* and homosexuality and may occasionally lead to violent sexual attacks. In most circumstances, a mild form of sexual inhibition is normal, so that sexuality does not disturb everyday social contact. Excessive sexuality, known in women as nymphomania and in men as satyriasis, may occur as a result of failure to establish a lasting satisfactory relationship. It may also be a symptom of *mania*, psychotic mental illness (see *Psychosis*) or, occasionally, excessive hormonal activity.

Vaginismus is a painful tightening of a woman's pelvic muscles around the vagina that prevents sexual intercourse. This usually has a psychological basis such as fear about sexual intercourse. Frigidity, a complete lack of sexual interest, may be associated with fear of pregnancy, *venereal disease* or pain, or with the belief that sexual intercourse is immoral. Failure of orgasm in women may be a mild form of frigidity but it may also indicate fatigue, illness or another minor disorder in a normally happy relationship.

Erection problems (impotence) may occur in a man for psychological reasons. Premature ejaculation of sperm frequently occurs in men when they are sexually inexperienced, anxious or if they feel guilty about sex.

Homosexuality is sexual attraction for someone of the same sex. In women it is known as lesbianism. It is a normal stage in the development of *sexuality* and many people maintain happy and contented homosexual relationships without any need for heterosexual intercourse. Some people are bisexual, having sexual relationships with both sexes. Variations in sexual behaviour become psychological problems only where they cause anxiety or guilt. Oral sex, anal sex and sex involving the use of slight pain (sadism or masochism) are common. In extreme forms such variations are abnormal and can be dangerous.

Incest is an illegal sexual relationship with a close relative, such as father with daughter, mother with son, or brother with sister. It is particularly likely to occur in social circumstances in which members of a family are forced into unusually close contact with one another.

Sexuality. The complicated association of natural instincts leading to the desire for sexual reproduction. Sexuality is specifically used to describe the psychological and physical responses of one person in sexual relation to another. This feeling of attraction and compatibility varies greatly between people and is modified by different circumstances. A child learns how to attract and respond to parents and friends before puberty. After puberty these subtle patterns are used with strangers and help to establish new friendships, some of which may be physically sexual, until a permanent relationship is formed that may lead to marriage.

The self-stimulation of sexual areas to produce an orgasm (*masturbation*) is a common and normal method of obtaining relief from the feeling of physical sexual tension when sexual intercourse is not possible. It starts during infancy and becomes more frequent at puberty. It can produce feelings of guilt if the child is reprimanded and can make the child feel that sexuality is in some way unhealthy or bad. This may distort normal sexual development in a child and lead to frigidity or impotence in an adult.

If a child's normal sexuality is frustrated, feelings of guilt and inhibition occur. These tend to prevent normal adult sexual development and leave the individual with underlying sexual desires that remain frustrated and in need of fulfilment. Various aspects of abnormal sexual development are discussed below.

Exhibitionism in young children is a form of infantile sexuality in which the child exhibits its genitals in order to attract a parent. In an adult male, it is an expression of his fear and dislike of women. A similar sexual gratification is sought by the voyeur, who observes a person of the opposite sex undressing, either in commercial strip-tease shows or through the window of a private house.

Fetishism originally described the worship of an object imbued with supernatural power. It is now used more commonly to refer to the sexual attraction to objects associated with sex. Fetishism, in certain cases, may be the only form in which sexual satisfaction can be attained, or it may simply be an aid to sexual activity.

Narcissism is a form of excessive self-love. It is a stage in the sexual development of all children which usually passes as the child progresses to more satisfying social relationships. If the stage persists, however, it may prevent the development of satisfactory adult relationships.

Pedophilia is a sexual love for children. Avoidance of the responsibilities of adult relationships may lead to misinterpretation of a simple, loving relationship with a child as an ideal sexual relationship. The child may respond with a similar love and this can cause the child to suffer emotional problems when the relationship is broken. In its extreme form, in which the child is molested sexually, it is illegal.

All serious problems due to failure of normal sexual development need skilled psychiatric care. Psychoanalysis may be needed to find the point at which normal development was frustrated, before any real help can be given.

Shingles (herpes zoster). A *herpes* virus related to *chickenpox* that affects parts of a cranial or spinal nerve and causes painful spots and blisters to erupt along the course of a peripheral nerve. Typically it affects the trunk of the body or the face. Symptoms include local pain, *malaise* and slight *fever* followed by red *rash* over the distribution of the nerve endings, which develops into clear blisters that become milky and then form scabs after three or four days. The pain is variable and may be intense. Complications can include eye problems, infection of the blisters, and pain in the nerve which may continue for several months after the disease itself has disappeared.

TREATMENT. Although mild forms of the illness clear without problems, a doctor should be consulted. A special antiviral drug applied to the skin at the onset of the illness will greatly help to reduce the severity of blistering and pain. When blisters are bursting, calamine lotion applied 2–3 times a day, antihistamine drugs to stop *itching*, and light cotton clothing will increase comfort. Pain-killing drugs and bed rest, a light, nutritious diet and adequate convalescence are usually required, as it may take a number of weeks before recovery is complete.

Sinusitis. Inflammation of the accessory nasal cavities which open into the main nasal passages. Symptoms are variable pain over the affected sinus, *catarrh* and possibly *fever*. Causes include *allergies*, *colds*, *catarrh*, *measles*, tooth infection and diving. Some people are predisposed to sinusitis because of inadequate drainage of the sinuses, which may be caused by a deviated nasal septum or by chronic rhinitis.

TREATMENT. Consult a doctor. Nose drops, steam inhalations, antihistamines, pain-killing drugs or antibiotics may be recommended.

Sleep-walking. Sleep-walking occurs most commonly between the ages of five and ten. It is not dangerous and the sleep-walker seems to retain normal cautiousness. Its causes are not clearly known, but underlying emotional insecurity or anxiety may be the cause in some children.

TREATMENT. Sleep-walking usually ceases naturally so there is no need for treatment. Take the child back to bed. There is no harm in waking a sleep-walker. Do not be anxious yourself as this will only worry the child.

Slipped disc. Each bone (vertebra) in the spine has a thick pad of fibrous tissue between it and the next one. This disc-shaped pad has a softer jelly-like centre. If the fibrous tissue tears, the softer centre can protrude to press on a nerve, and so cause pain and loss of sensation, as in *sciatica*.

TREATMENT. The protrusion eventually diminishes in size if the patient rests. Antirheumatic drugs may help this process. Manipulation or stretching the spine (traction) causes a change in direction of the protrusion and may relieve pressure on the nerve.

Smallpox (variola). Until recently this was a very serious virus infection, characterized by the appearance of pustules after an incubation of up to two weeks. Since January 1st, 1980 the World Health Organization has declared the world free of this disease and vaccination is no longer required.

Smear test (Papanicolaou smear). In the course of a normal vaginal examination a few cells are removed from the surface of the cervix of the womb so that they can be examined under a microscope. This examination detects whether they are normal or whether they show signs of infection, abnormalities not due to cancer, or changes that may be early indications of *cancer*. If the test is performed about once a year, precancerous cells can be detected and highly effective treatment can be given before cancer develops.

Smoking. The effects of smoking on health are numerous. Those who smoke 25 cigarettes a day have a death rate from chronic *bronchitis* that is 20 times greater than non-smokers. *Cancer* of the lung kills one man in seven in the 55–60 age group. Smoking increases the dangers of *heart attack* and *arteriosclerosis*, doubles the risk of *cancer* of the bladder and is also a significant factor in some forms of *blindness*, *gingivitis*, and peptic *ulcers*. In women, smoking increases the probability of *stillbirth* and *miscarriage*, and the birth weight of babies born to women who smoke is lower than average.
TREATMENT. Discuss the habit with a doctor. To stop smoking requires determination. The doctor may recommend some drugs that can help. The physical withdrawal takes about two weeks, during which time craving may become severe. After two weeks any further symptoms are probably psychological in origin.

Snoring. Noisy breathing while asleep. It may be caused by *catarrh*, enlarged *adenoids* or a deviated nasal septum. For most people, however, it is simply the result of sleeping on the back with the mouth open which causes vibration of the back of the palate.

Sore throat. A sore throat can occur with any infection of the respiratory tract. It may also be caused by *smoking* or by breathing in a smoky atmosphere. If the soreness persists for more than 12 hours, if it becomes worse, or if it is associated with *fever*, it may be a symptom of *influenza, tonsillitis, infectious mononucleosis*, or a throat infection caused by a virus or by bacteria such as streptococci (see *Strep throat*). Throat infections are easily transmitted, and a persistent sore throat should be reported to a doctor.
TREATMENT. When the soreness is first noticed, gargle with soluble aspirin in warm water and swallow. Avoid crowded places so that the disease does not spread. See also *Diphtheria* and CHART OF WHAT TO DO: Sore throat, p.95.

Spina bifida. This is a congenital deformity of the lower part of the spine due to failure of the vertebrae to join. It may be so slight that it is noticed only on an X-ray, or so severe that none of the tissues over the lower part of the back have joined and the covering of the spinal cord is exposed. The severe form is often associated with hydrocephalus, a condition in which the brain of the child swells because the normal circulation of its fluid is blocked. As the brain swells, the skull also increases in size. The causes of these congenital abnormalities are not known. Spina bifida can often be detected by special tests in early pregnancy. In the mild form there may be no symptoms. *Paralysis* of the legs and bladder may occur in the severe form and *meningitis* may develop because the membranes surrounding the spinal cord are exposed.

Spondylitis and spondylosis. Spondylitis is an inflammation of the vertebrae, most commonly due to a rheumatic disorder, ankylosing spondylitis (*poker back*), that more usually affects young men than women. Spondylosis, a degenerative condition, is osteo*arthritis* of the spine. Both conditions may cause stiffness, pain and pressure on the nerves, and neuritis.
TREATMENT. Antirheumatic drugs and, occasionally, spinal braces will help.

Sprain. An injury to the ligaments around a joint, caused by a violent, sudden movement. It usually affects the ankle or the wrist. The symptoms are pain, swelling and an inability to move the joint.
TREATMENT. Treat as a *fracture* until the injury has been examined by a doctor. See also FIRST AID: Sprain, p.42.

Stiff neck. A symptom of muscle strain, but if persistent may indicate *rheumatism, fibrositis,* or possibly a *slipped disc.*
TREATMENT. Warmth on the affected area and massage may relieve the stiffness. If it persists, consult a doctor. If stiff neck is accompanied by *headache, fever* and dislike of bright lights, a doctor must be consulted at once.

Stillbirth. A baby that is born dead after the 28th week of pregnancy is described as stillborn. Death may be caused by congenital abnormalities, prolonged and difficult labour, or maternal illness such as high *blood pressure* or untreated *syphilis.* An unusually premature birth may cause a baby to be stillborn, but good antenatal care reduces the chances of this happening.

Stomach ache. A diffuse abdominal discomfort, seldom severe enough to cause pain or interfere with normal work. It is usually associated with *indigestion.* See also *Abdominal pain, Gastritis, Flatulence, Nausea* and CHART OF WHAT TO DO: Stomach ache, p.92.

Stone in kidney. Stones may be formed from excess salts and uric acid. They are usually caused by a lack of fluid in hot climates, *gout,* infection, or congenital abnormalities. There are often no symptoms unless the stone moves and causes an obstruction. In such cases *colic,* severe *backache,* spasmodic pain in the groin, *vomiting,* sweating, and frequent *urination* with evidence of blood in the *urine* may occur.
TREATMENT. Call a doctor as soon as symptoms develop. Strong pain-killing and antispasm drugs may be required. An intravenous pyelogram (see *Kidney disorders*) shows the stone's position. It may be possible to remove the stone through the bladder, or an abdominal operation may be necessary.

Strep throat. An infection of the throat by a strain of streptococcus bacteria. The symptoms include marked inflammation, pain on swallowing, and *fever*. Infections of this type spread easily and if left untreated may lead to serious conditions elsewhere in the body. See also *Nephritis, Rheumatic fever, Scarlet fever, Sore throat* and *Tonsillitis*.

TREATMENT. Consult a doctor as soon as possible. Antibiotic therapy is usually required. Gargling with antiseptic mouth wash may relieve the inflammation.

Stroke. A problem affecting the brain and causing symptoms elsewhere in the body. The brain is damaged by hemorrhage, blockage of an artery due to *embolus, thrombosis* or *arteriosclerosis*. The symptoms indicate which part of the brain has been damaged. A stroke may cause momentary weakness, numbness, disordered speech or double vision, accompanied by some degree of *paralysis*, and may be followed by complete recovery. A serious stroke may result in *paralysis* of half the body (hemiplegia) or death.

TREATMENT. Call a doctor or ambulance immediately. Do not give the patient anything to drink. Lie the patient in the recovery position (see LIFE-SAVING: Recovery position, p.18) and continue to check for breathing and pulse (see LIFE-SAVING: Checking for breathing and pulse, p.12) until the ambulance arrives.

Sty. A sty is an infected hair follicle in the eyelid. It often occurs in children, and may be associated with *conjunctivitis*.

TREATMENT. See FIRST AID: Sty, p.43.

Synovitis. An inflammation or infection of the membranes that produce synovial fluid. These membranes and their synovial fluid surround tendons, joints, and other places where friction occurs. Inflammation of these places may also be described as *tenosynovitis, capsulitis* or *bursitis*, and occurs because of injuries or strains, infections, or diseases such as rheumatoid *arthritis*. Symptoms include pain, local tenderness and swelling, and difficulties in movement.

TREATMENT. The affected joint or limb should be rested, using a sling or splint if necessary. Antibiotics, aspirin, antirheumatic drugs, or injection of corticosteroid drugs may be required, following a doctor's advice.

Syphilis. The most serious of *venereal diseases*, syphilis is caused by the organism Treponema pallidum, usually transmitted through sexual intercourse. The chief symptom of the primary stage is *chancre* which appears within three weeks of contracting the disease. The second stage, which occurs six or eight weeks later, is indicated by a mild *fever*, a *rash* over the body, swollen lymph glands, *sore throat* and *headache*. The third stage may not occur for ten to 15 years. Swellings in any tissue may develop and interfere with the normal workings of the body. The final stage involves the nervous system and causes the condition known as general paralysis of the insane, symptoms of which include loss of sensation in the legs, a staggering gait and ulceration of the skin.

TREATMENT. The disease is highly contagious in the early stages and sexual intercourse must be avoided completely. Penicillin is curative in adequate doses but careful examination must be carried out over the following few years to ensure that the disease has been killed.

T

Teething. Some babies are born with teeth and others do not produce them until they are more than one year old. Teething usually causes little trouble apart from occasional slight irritation and apparent discomfort. A teething ring may help this. Children usually have all their milk teeth by the age of 30 months and start losing them, when the permanent teeth arrive, from the age of about six years.

Tenosynovitis. Inflammation of the sheath of a tendon, causing swelling and pain when the tendon is moved. In certain cases a grating sensation accompanies movement.
TREATMENT. The inflammation will usually disappear with rest, but in severe cases it may be necessary to drain the fluid from the tendon sheath. Treatment with antirheumatic and corticosteroid drugs is sometimes necessary.

Tetanus (lockjaw). Disease marked by painful spasms of the muscles of the jaw or other parts of the body. They are caused by the
[H] tetanus bacillus, which grows at the site of a wound and produces a toxin that causes the muscles to move with reflex spasms. These symptoms develop several days or weeks after the wound has become infected. The spasms are exhausting and, if they affect the respiratory muscles, may cause asphyxia. They are usually associated with *fever* and the disease is often fatal.
TREATMENT. Proper medical attention must be given to dirty wounds. Antitetanus serum and antibiotics are required to prevent the development of the disease. *Immunization* is recommended and a booster is required from time to time.

Thrombosis. This occurs when a blood clot (thrombus) forms in part of the circulation and obstructs the blood flow. Throm-
[icon] bosis is likely to occur in blood vessel diseases such as *arteriosclerosis*, *phlebitis*, and *varicose veins*, or as a side-effect of *smoking* or use of the pill (see *Contraception*). Any blood clotting is known as thrombosis and this is not necessarily pathological. Thrombosis of small veins always occurs around the site of an injury or infection.
A deep vein thrombosis usually occurs in the large veins deep in the muscles of the calf, thigh, or pelvis. It may occur after childbirth or an operation. The first signs may be ankle swelling or calf tenderness. If a piece of thrombus breaks off it forms an *embolus*. A superficial venous thrombosis may occur in *phlebitis*. An arterial thrombosis is always serious. Coronary thrombosis leads to a *heart attack*. Thrombosis in an arteriosclerotic leg can lead to *gangrene*. In the brain a thrombosis causes a *stroke*.
TREATMENT. Thrombosis may be prevented by starting to take physical activity as soon as possible after an operation or, in certain cases, by the use of anticoagulant drugs. A deep vein thrombosis also requires treatment with anticoagulants, but thrombophlebitis can be treated successfully with local heat and antirheumatic or pain-killing drugs if necessary.

Thumb sucking. Thumb sucking is normal in most newborn babies, and soon stops. It is likely to return at the age of about six months and is a habit that seems to comfort and reassure a child and often helps with sleep. It usually ceases by the age of four or five.

Thyroid problems. The thyroid gland lies in front of the windpipe (trachea) in the neck. Hormones from the thyroid, particularly thyroxine, control the speed of activity (metabolism) of the cells of the body.

Over-production of thyroxine is known as hyperthyroidism. Symptoms include *palpitations*, sweating, large appetite but loss of weight, sometimes *diarrhea* and *menstrual disorders*, protruding eyes, and trembling hands. A lack of thyroxine (hypothyroidism or myxedema) sometimes occurs after treatment for hyperthyroidism, but it is also associated with increasing age and thyroid failure. Babies born with too little thyroxine may suffer from cretinism, causing mental retardation. Symptoms of hypothyroidism include lethargy, mental slowing, complaints of cold, hair falling out and coarsening of the skin.

TREATMENT. For hyperthyroidism, younger patients are given pills to reduce thyroid activity. This may be followed by an operation to remove part of the thyroid gland. Older patients are usually treated with radioactive iodine. This is safe but it may eventually lead to hypothyroidism. For hypothyroidism, consult a doctor, who will usually give thyroxine tablets.

Tinea (ringworm). A fungus infection of the skin. It is usually contracted in communal wash-places such as school and sports club shower-rooms and swimming pools, from contaminated damp towels and wet floors. Occasionally animal ringworm is caught from close contact with sheep, cattle, dogs or cats. Tinea may infect the creases between the toes (*athlete's foot*), the groin, the armpits, the nails and, occasionally, the scalp. Animal ringworm tends to cause large rings, with slightly raised edges, anywhere on the skin. Normally ringworm is a mildly irritating red patch which becomes sore when moist.

TREATMENT. Antifungal creams and powders usually cure athlete's foot but other areas may need more specific medical attention. Infection of the nails requires prolonged therapy with antifungal drugs.

Toenail, ingrowing. This usually affects the big toes and is often caused by pressure from tight shoes and incorrect nail-cutting. The ingrowing nail cuts into the side of the toe forming a fissure which may become infected, especially when there is a lack of cleanliness.

TREATMENT. Infection should be treated by applying strips of gauze soaked in antiseptic liquid to the side of the nail, but if it continues, consult a doctor. Prevent recurrences by cutting the nails so that the corners do not stick into the skin.

Tonsillitis. An inflammation due to infection of the lymphatic tissue at the back of the mouth (tonsils). With the *adenoids* in the nose the tonsils protect the throat and lungs from infecting organisms that may enter through the mouth and nose. They help to establish immunity to common infective agents and are most active in childhood, when many infections are encountered for the first time. Large tonsils are not abnormal at this age. If the tonsils are no longer able to cope with infections they may become inflamed and tonsillitis will occur. The symptoms of this are a *sore throat*, a *fever* and persistent *malaise*. Recurrent attacks of tonsillitis, or a chronic infection lasting several years, may be indications for their removal (tonsillectomy). See also *Strep throat*.

TREATMENT. A doctor must be consulted. Gargle with soluble

aspirin in warm water and swallow it. Antiseptic mouth washes and throat lozenges also help. In more serious cases the doctor may use antibiotics to combat the infection.

Toothache. Pain in or around a tooth, which may be so severe that it appears to affect the whole side of the jaw. It may be caused by an infection in the tooth itself due to food that has lodged in a cavity or it may be due to a *gumboil* around the base of the tooth. In children toothache may be caused by a secondary tooth pushing at the root of a milk tooth that is due to fall. TREATMENT. Dental treatment is required in most cases, and medical advice may also be required for treatment of a gumboil. Toothache is most easily prevented by dental care in the home and by regular visits to a dentist. See FIRST AID: Dental problems, p.26

Tracheitis. An inflammation of the trachea, associated with *laryngitis* and *bronchitis*. Symptoms include a *cough* that causes pain behind the upper part of the breastbone and sometimes a mild *fever*. TREATMENT. Steam inhalations, cough mixtures and a warm, humid room may relieve the symptoms until recovery. If the inflammation persists or becomes too uncomfortable, a doctor should be consulted. The patient must stop *smoking*.

Traveller's diarrhea. This is a general name for intestinal disorders that occur following a change in country, climate and diet. The usual causes are an unfamiliar diet, excessive intake of fruit, especially if this is not carefully washed, unusually large quantities of alcohol, particularly wine, inadequate sanitation, or true intestinal infections. TREATMENT. Do not drink water that has not been boiled or sterilized: drinking water can be bought in many countries. Take care with alcohol and dietary excess and avoid precooked foods and unwashed and unpeeled fruit. Proprietary drugs such as Loperamide may help. During the attack itself, drink plenty of fluids, if necessary with extra salt, to prevent dehydration. Use antidiarrheal medicines recommended by a doctor. If severe *diarrhea* persists for more than 24 hours, particularly if associated with a *fever* or dehydration, consult a doctor.

Travel sickness. Common among children, particularly those who develop *migraine*; occurs frequently on the sea, in cars and buses, and less frequently in trains or planes. Caused by swaying movement affecting the organ of balance in the ear. TREATMENT. If a child is known to be travel sick, give antinauseant drugs, obtainable from your pharmacist, the night before and on the morning of a long journey. Ensure that meals are small in volume and easily digestible, and that not too much fluid is drunk at once; small drinks, however, should be given frequently. Let the child sleep if possible. See also FIRST AID: Travel sickness, p.43

Tuberculosis. A bacterial infection, caused by Mycobacterium bacteria, that may affect the respiratory system, gastrointestinal and urogenital tracts, the nervous system, joints and bones, or the skin. The disease may be carried by people, cattle or birds. Tuberculosis develops gradually, causing symptoms of *malaise, fever,* loss of weight and often a *cough.* The infection may also remain dormant for long periods, causing the symptoms to recur from time to time as the disease progresses.

TREATMENT. Drugs are effective in most cases but treatment may have to continue for up to two years. Contacts require chest X-rays and BCG vaccination. *Immunization* protects those who have not been in contact with the disease.

Tumour. A lump or swelling in the body tissues. It may be due to an infection such as an *abscess*, to local damage such as a bruise or to an abnormal growth of body tissue. This abnormal growth may be due to *cancer* or it may be a benign growth such as a lipoma, *polyp* or a fibrous tissue swelling (fibroma).

TREATMENT. There are many types of tumour, so each must be diagnosed carefully for the appropriate treatment. If you find an abnormal swelling you should consult a doctor. Tumours in the breast may be detected by monthly examination with the flat of the hand: see *Breast examination*.

Typhoid (enteric fever). An infection, due to bacteria of the Salmonella genus, that is spread by contaminated water, milk and food. Symptoms include the gradual onset of *fever, headache, constipation, cough*, and scattered pink spots on the trunk, and usually appear within three weeks of contracting the disease. Complications include intestinal hemorrhage and perforation of the bowel causing *peritonitis*.

TREATMENT. Isolation in a hospital is required for treatment with antibiotics. Examination of the feces is necessary to ensure that the disease has been cured. *Immunization* against typhoid is available.

Typhus. A group of diseases carried by *lice*, ticks and fleas. Symptoms appear abruptly a few days to three weeks after being bitten. There is usually a large red scab at the site of the bite. This is followed by a high *fever*, severe *headache, delirium*, the appearance of purple spots on the trunk and limbs, and severe illness lasting for seven to ten days.

TREATMENT. The most common form of typhus is associated with unhygienic conditions and may be prevented by adequate sanitation and cleanliness. *Immunization* is temporarily effective. Hospital treatment with antibiotics is required.

U

Ulcer. A peptic ulcer occurs because excess acid erodes the wall of the stomach or the duodenum. Many factors may contribute to this damage, usually by affecting the normally protective lining of the stomach. An acute ulcer may be caused in this way by alcohol, aspirin, antirheumatic or corticosteroid drugs, or by acute stress resulting from an operation or from burns. Chronic ulcers occur more often in middle-aged men than women. Most affect the duodenum and are probably influenced by long-term stress, excessive *alcohol* consumption and *smoking*. Symptoms include attacks of upper *abdominal pain*, occurring about two hours after a meal and often accompanied by *heartburn, nausea* and *vomiting*. These may be relieved by milk and antacids.

TREATMENT. Medical treatment with antacids and drugs helps to reduce acid secretion, as does a diet of small, regular, bland meals. Smoking and alcohol and foods that aggravate the stomach, such as spiced or fried foods, should all be avoided. Surgery is indicated if other treatment fails, if there is evidence of bleeding, if the ulcer perforates the stomach lining, or if extreme scarring causes obstruction.

Ulcer, mouth. A small blister that commonly occurs on the side or tip of the tongue and ruptures to form a small painful spot. The ulcer is usually white with an inflamed rim. Ulcers may occur because of *indigestion*, irritation of the tongue by the rough surface of a tooth, or because of a *cold*.
TREATMENT. A mouth wash reduces the inflammation and ulcers normally heal rapidly without further treatment. If necessary a proprietary ointment may be used. See also FIRST AID: Dental problems, p.26.

Urination, frequent. This may be a symptom of *cystitis*, particularly if it occurs with pain, or of *anxiety* or *diabetes*. It may also occur in *pregnancy* because of pressure on the bladder by the growing fetus. In an older woman it may be caused by *fibroids* or *prolapse of the womb*. If frequent urination persists with no obvious cause for more than few days, a doctor should be consulted. See *Prostate problems* and CHART OF WHAT TO DO: Increased urination, p.99.

Urine, blood in (hematuria). This may be a symptom of *cystitis* or *prostate problems* if it is associated with pain on urination, or of *nephritis* or *pyelonephritis* if there is also *backache* and *fever*. Growths or *stones in the kidney* or bladder may cause painless hematuria.
TREATMENT. Consult a doctor as soon as possible, taking a sample of urine with you for examination.

Urine, discoloration of. The urine is naturally darker in the morning, during a fever and if one is dehydrated. It is very dark in some illnesses such as *jaundice*, blood in the urine (see previous entry), and it may also be darkened by some drugs. Sometimes a milky discoloration occurs due to the crystallization of salts in concentrated urine, but this is not serious. The smell of urine varies with concentration and diet, but a strong fishy smell is often associated with *cystitis* and urinary infections.
TREATMENT. If the urine appears unusually dark or cloudy, increase the amount of fluids drunk. If the discoloration or strange smell persists, consult a doctor for advice, taking a sample of the urine for examination.

Urine, retention of. The inability to urinate, despite feeling the need to do so, may indicate *prostate problems* or *cystitis*. It may also be a sign of a neurological problem such as a *stroke*. It is common after an operation, particularly a gynecological one, in which local bruising causes this temporary reaction.
TREATMENT. A hot bath or the sound of running water may help urination to occur. Pain-killing drugs may be useful. If these measures fail, consult a doctor. Hospital admission may be required for a tube (catheter) to be passed into the bladder to drain the urine. See also FIRST AID: Urine, unable to pass, p.44.

V

Vaginal bleeding. Bleeding from the vagina is normal if it is due to *periods*. Abnormal, unexpected bleeding may be associated with *menstrual disorders*, the *menopause* or *contraception*, particularly if the contraceptive pill or an intrauterine device is used. If a woman is pregnant, bleeding probably indicates a threatened *miscarriage*. In all cases unusual bleeding should be reported to a doctor, particularly if it occurs after the menopause, and should be done as soon as possible if the bleeding is severe.

Vaginal discharge. The normal vaginal secretion varies within the menstrual cycle, increasing at the time of ovulation and increasing again before and just after menstruation. The amount of discharge varies greatly from woman to woman and is often increased by sexual stimulation, the *contraceptive* pill, or *anxiety.* An abnormal discharge (*vaginitis*), usually indicated by irritation, slight bleeding or unpleasant smell, may be a sign of vaginal, cervical or uterine infections.

Vaginitis. An infection of the vagina. It may be a mild type of infection caused by a variety of organisms including the fungus causing *moniliasis* (thrush). Monilial vaginitis may also be associated with *pregnancy* or with the use of the *contraceptive* pill. It may also occur in *diabetes,* or as a result of using antibiotics or corticosteroid drugs, or from douching with chemicals that are too strong. Trichomoniasis is a form of vaginitis caused by minute moving parasites that may live in the vagina. Symptoms are not always obvious but they usually cause discharge when the vaginal wall is disturbed by sexual intercourse, menstruation or an illness. Trichomoniasis and moniliasis may also cause the vulva to itch and to discharge profusely, sometimes with slight bleeding.
TREATMENT. The condition must be reported to a doctor for a correct diagnosis. Drugs are usually given in the form of pessaries or creams to put in the vagina. Trichomoniasis also responds to drugs taken by mouth. In trichomoniasis and moniliasis both sexual partners should be treated.

Varicose veins. These are distorted, dilated veins usually found in the legs. They may be caused by damage to the valves following *thrombosis* or pregnancy or they may be due to a congenital defect in the valves. The pressure of blood, without the regulating effect of the valves, causes the veins to swell, to lose their elasticity and finally to remain dilated. Symptoms include aching legs, swelling and ulceration at the ankles, *eczema,* and sometimes *thrombosis.*
TREATMENT. Elastic stockings to support the veins and sitting with the legs raised may both help. An injection into the veins may be given to make them collapse completely. Six weeks' firm bandaging is required after this injection to make sure that the walls of the veins stick to each other. An operation to remove a vein or to cut it in various places to prevent back-pressure in the damaged vein may be required. If a varicose vein bursts, see FIRST AID: Bleeding, p.21.

Venereal diseases (sexually transmitted diseases). *Gonorrhea* and *syphilis* are commonly thought to be the main diseases caught by sexual contact, but there are several others including some that are only sometimes sexually transmitted. See *A.I.D.S., Chancroid, Granuloma inguinale, Herpes genitalis, Lice, Lymphogranuloma venereum, Moniliasis, Nonspecific urethritis, Scabies, Vaginitis* (trichomoniasis) and *Verrucas and warts.*

Verrucas and warts. Small tumours of the skin caused by a virus infection. Warts and verrucas are commonest in children aged between eight and 12 and occur most commonly as small growths on the hands but also on the face and the soles of the feet. In adults they may be sexually transmitted on the penis and vulva. The term verruca is commonly used for a wart on the sole of the foot (plantar wart), where pressure on it is painful. Most warts disappear spontaneously within a year without treatment.

TREATMENT. Consult a doctor. If necessary warts can be removed by cutting them out, by slowly burning them with acid, or by freezing them with carbon dioxide snow.

Vitamins. Essential substances, small amounts of which are required in the diet for the normal working of the body. They are classified in two main groups: those that dissolve in fat and those that dissolve in water.

Vitamin A. A fat-soluble vitamin found in liver, cod liver oil, butter and eggs. It is necessary for vision in poor light and for a healthy skin. Deficiency leads to night blindness and dry skin. An excess may cause liver damage, drowsiness and headache.

Vitamin B$_1$ (thiamin). A water-soluble vitamin found in milk, eggs, wholewheat bread and fruit. It is necessary for the metabolism of carbohydrates. Deficiency leads to beri-beri, either wet with *heart failure* or dry with *polyneuritis*.

Vitamin B$_2$ (riboflavin). A water-soluble vitamin found in milk, liver, yeast, kidney and eggs, necessary for releasing energy from food. Deficiency, which is rare, causes soreness at the corners of the mouth.

Nicotinic acid (niacin). A water-soluble vitamin of the B group, found in bread, milk, vegetables and meat. It is important for preventing the skin condition pellagra.

Vitamin B$_6$ (pyridoxin). A water-soluble vitamin found in most foods, particularly meat, eggs, fish and flour. It is necessary for the formation of body protein. Symptoms of deficiency are rare, but may include *anemia*.

Vitamin B$_{12}$. A water-soluble vitamin found in liver, eggs and cheese, important for normal blood production and healthy nerve tissue. Deficiency leads to pernicious *anemia* and *polyneuritis*.

Folic acid. A water-soluble vitamin found in liver, kidney and leaf vegetables, required for normal blood production. Deficiency leads to *anemia*.

Pantothenic acid and biotin. Water-soluble vitamins found in most foods, used in the formation of body fats. Deficiency does not occur.

Vitamin C (ascorbic acid). A water-soluble vitamin found in green vegetables, fruit and potatoes. It is necessary to keep body tissues adherent to each other. Deficiency leads to scurvy, in which the tissues tend to disintegrate.

Vitamin D. A fat-soluble vitamin found in cod liver oil, fatty fish, eggs, milk and butter. It is needed to maintain the calcium level in blood and bone. Deficiency leads to *rickets* and osteomalacia, caused by softening of the bone. An excess causes too much calcium to be absorbed and this can damage kidney tissue, particularly of children, and occasionally other parts of the body such as the tendons.

Vitamin E. A fat-soluble vitamin found in most foods, particularly vegetable oils, eggs and flour. Its value is uncertain.

Vitamin K. A fat-soluble vitamin found in leaf vegetables, pulses and cereals. It is synthesized in the intestine, and is required for the normal clotting mechanisms of the blood. Deficiency rarely occurs except with severe *liver disease*, *cirrhosis*, or following the use of certain drugs.

Vomiting. May be caused by *gastric 'flu, food poisoning, travel* sickness, nausea, infectious *hepatitis, pregnancy,* the use of oral *contraception,* gastrointestinal obstruction, dietary or alcohol excess, or an overdose of medically prescribed drugs. It may also be associated with *anorexia nervosa, migraine,* or *abdominal pain* and *diarrhea.*

TREATMENT. Treatment must be directed at the cause, but it will help to take sips of water, suck ice cubes, lie down and keep warm. Consult a doctor if vomiting occurs as frequently as once or twice an hour for more than four hours, if it is associated with pain, or if it continues for more than a day. See also FIRST AID: Vomiting, p.44 and CHART OF WHAT TO DO: Vomiting, p.93.

Vomiting, in babies. Many babies regurgitate after a feed. This is not harmful and may be a sign of contentment. Occasionally an older baby vomits regularly after a meal but gains weight and is clearly well. This too is a habit, often in a lively, cheerful baby. Vomiting may occur during a *cold* if mucus is swallowed and then vomited, or following a severe coughing bout, particularly with *whooping cough.* It may also occur as a part of a generalized illness associated with *fever,* such as a middle ear infection (*otitis media*), or with *diarrhea.* If it is caused by intestinal obstruction, *colic* and abdominal swelling will also be apparent. Rarely, vomiting may indicate an allergy to cow's milk.

TREATMENT. Decide whether the vomiting is due to regurgitation or whether it is associated with a *cold* or more serious problem. Dehydration, usually due to vomiting associated with *diarrhea,* is a potential danger. Generalized infections and intestinal obstructions need rapid medical attention. Less serious vomiting is treated by resting the stomach. Stop meals and give small amounts of water every hour and increase this quantity only when the vomiting has stopped. As soon as the baby has started to drink properly, half-strength milk and then solids can be given. See also FIRST AID: Dehydration, p.26.

Vulvitis. An inflammation of the vulva, the outer part of the female genitals at the entrance to the vagina. It may be associated with *vaginitis, herpes genitalis,* an infection of lubricating glands causing abscesses (Bartholin's abscess), or with rubbing from pads or clothes that are too tight.

TREATMENT. Consult a doctor. If the area is very sore and uncomfortable a cold compress will often relieve the symptoms. If the inflammation is painful, drugs such as aspirin may be used until further treatment is started.

W

Water on the knee. A knee swollen by excess fluid in the joint cavity under the kneecap. It may be caused by an injury to the knee, a torn *cartilage, arthritis* or *synovitis.*

TREATMENT. Tie a firm elastic crepe bandage around the knee when it is straight and rest the knee as much as possible. Aspirin and antirheumatic drugs sometimes help. If the symptoms persist exercises are necessary to keep thigh muscles strong. In all cases a doctor should be consulted.

Wax. Ear wax is a sticky, orange-brown secretion from the external tube of the ear which may block it and cause irritation or *deafness.*

TREATMENT. Consult a doctor. Do not attempt to extract a plug of wax yourself as you risk pushing it farther in and possibly damaging the eardrum.

Whitlow. An infection around the nails at the ends of the fingers or toes. The symptoms include pain and swelling followed by the formation of pus. It is commonly caused by nail-biting or by working with the hands in hot water or in unhygienic conditions. It may also be due to *moniliasis* (candidiasis).
TREATMENT. If the infection is severe, a minor operation under local anesthetic is required to open and clean the wound. Antifungal creams will prevent moniliasis.

Whooping cough (pertussis). A bacterial infection, particularly dangerous to children. The incubation period is usually about ten days and the disease is infectious for about three weeks. Symptoms include *catarrh* with mild *fever* at the onset followed by a *cough* that increases in severity. The cough starts with a spasm and ends with a sharp intake of breath, the whoop. A prolonged coughing spell is often followed by *vomiting*. Whooping cough may last up to five or six weeks and may cause *nosebleeds*, debility and *insomnia*. Complications include *encephalitis, pneumonia, sinusitis* and *otitis media*.
TREATMENT. Antibiotics given in the early stages may help. No effective cough mixture is available. Bed rest, sedation at night, sufficient fluid to drink and frequent light meals help to sustain the patient through the course of the disease. Patients should be observed carefully for complications.
Quarantine: 21 days after last contact with the disease. See also *Immunization*.

Wind. Air swallowing occurs naturally in babies during feeding. It is increased by too small a hole in the nipple. A baby likes to be cuddled and played with after a feed and this is the time when excess wind may be burped up. See also *Colic*.

Worms. Parasitic worms are commonly transmitted by contaminated food or water or by the bites of certain animals or insects.
There are two main groups of parasitic worms. (1) The roundworms such as ascaris, enterobius (pinworm), and trichuris (whipworm) infest the intestine. The Filarioidea invade body tissues, causing filariasis. (2) The flatworms include flukes, which invade the body tissues to form cysts, and tapeworms, which usually inhabit the intestine.
TREATMENT. A diagnosis is usually made by finding intestinal worms in the feces. They sometimes cause intestinal pain or diarrhea and may cause listlessness. A doctor may prescribe medication to kill the worms. Infection of the body tissues requires special investigation and treatment.

Y

Yellow fever. A virus infection carried by mosquitoes. It occurs particularly in central Africa and parts of South America. The symptoms of *fever, vomiting*, dehydration, muscle pains and *jaundice* appear within a week of being bitten.
TREATMENT. *Immunization* provides protection in areas where yellow fever is endemic. There is no specific treatment for those who suffer from the disease, but rest, fluid replacement and a nutritious liquid diet, supplemented with vitamin K and calcium gluconate, help to sustain the patient through the course of the illness.

Medicinal drugs

Treatment with drugs is one of the most important areas of modern medicine, but also one about which the lay person knows least. For practical purposes different drugs are classified into types, according to their functions or general characteristics, and some features of these types, listed in alphabetical order, are described in the following pages.

Some drugs, such as aspirin and many antihistamines, can be bought from a pharmacist without a doctor's prescription. But most drugs need a prescription, and some dangerous ones such as morphine and amphetamine are under strict legal control.

Caution: Many drugs may slow physical reactions and cause drowsiness. Sleeping pills, tranquillizers and many others may have an effect for up to 24 hours after they are taken, although this may not be noticeable; this effect is increased by alcohol. Great care must therefore be taken when driving or using moving machinery. Your doctor should warn you of this and the pharmacist may label the drug container with a cautionary notice.

Anesthetics
General anesthetics are given before major surgery is carried out. A premedication injection is usually given before a general anesthetic. It acts as a relaxant with a mild sedative effect; it also dries the mouth. Local anesthetics may be injected, to numb a nerve or an area of skin, or sprayed or applied locally to the area to be anesthetized. Occasionally an allergic reaction may occur.

Antacids
Antacids may be alkalis used to neutralize stomach acids or drugs that reduce stomach acid secretion. Some preparations combine both sorts. Overdosage may cause a dry mouth and drowsiness.

Antiallergic drugs
These are the antihistamines, corticosteroid drugs and chromolyn sodium (Intal). These can be used in eye drops, in nasal and bronchial sprays, or as powders that are inhaled.

Antibiotics
Antibiotics comprise several groups of drugs that can kill bacteria. The use of antibiotics, however, may be hazardous. Excessive use of antibiotics encourages the development of resistant strains of bacteria and may also lead to an increased likelihood of allergic reactions. Particular infections often require specific antibiotics. Some of the more toxic antibiotics are safe to use on the skin but should not be taken internally.

Anticoagulants
Anticoagulants are drugs that interfere with the normal clotting of the blood and reduce the chances of thrombosis. They are used after deep vein and coronary thrombosis and in some forms of heart and gynecological surgery in which

the hazards of venous and arterial thrombosis are increased.

Anticonvulsant drugs
Anticonvulsants control epilepsy, and treatment with them usually continues for many years. Occasionally allergic reactions occur but, on the whole, these drugs are considered safe.

Antidepressants
Antidepressants work within the brain to alter the patient's mood. They may take two to three weeks to produce an effect, and the course of treatment should continue for several weeks after this. Apart from stimulant drugs such as amphetamine, there are two main groups of antidepressants. One group, the most commonly prescribed, benefits those who wake too early and suffer depression and anxiety at the beginning of the day. These may also cause dryness in the mouth, constipation and slight drowsiness. The other group, the mono-amine oxidase inhibitors (MAOI), may help those who sleep normally but suffer depression all day. This group of drugs may cause adverse reactions to certain foods such as cheese, yeast or meat extracts, broad beans, yogurt, alcohol and sometimes to other drugs, particularly pain-killers. Tranquillizers are often used in combination with antidepressants because anxiety is frequently associated with depression.

Antidiabetic drugs
Antidiabetic drugs are taken to replace or to stimulate the production of insulin. Excessive amounts may cause faintness, dizziness and sometimes coma due to hypoglycemia. Insulin is the most common drug used in the treatment of severe diabetes but can be given only by injection. It is prepared synthetically or from the pancreas of pigs or cattle; in rare cases the latter types may cause an allergic reaction. Simple preparations or slow-release preparations act for varying lengths of time. The dose has to be carefully calculated according to the patient's requirements.

Antidiarrheal drugs
The most common preparation used to treat diarrhea is kaolin which is sometimes combined with a small amount of morphine. The morphine group, including codeine, has a direct constipating effect on the bowel. Some types of antispasmodic drug (see below) may be obtained without a prescription and these are frequently used by vacationers to control traveller's diarrhea. Antibiotics may be used in some severe infections.

Antifungal drugs
Antifungal drugs are used in the treatment of moniliasis and tinea infections such as thrush and athlete's foot. Antifungals are usually applied directly to the affected area or membranes as creams, ointments or pessaries.

Antihistamines
This group of drugs is used in the treatment of allergies, asthma, insect bites and urticaria. They also act to prevent

motion sickness and may be used as sedatives for children. They occasionally cause unexpected stimulation or over-sedation and can be dangerous if taken before driving or using machinery. They can cause serious drowsiness if taken at the same time as alcohol.

Antimalarial drugs
Antimalarial drugs must be taken regularly when entering a malarious region and their use must be continued for at least a month after leaving the area. Different antimalarial types are designed to be taken either daily or weekly, depending on the kind of drug. If the disease is caught, specific drugs such as quinine or chloroquine may be required.

Antinausea and antiemetic drugs
Antihistamines and many of the major tranquillizer drugs have antinausea effects. Their use is not to be recommended during pregnancy because they may cause fetal damage. Particular care should be used if they are taken when driving. Alcohol should not be consumed when taking these drugs.

Anti-Parkinsonian drugs
These include levodopa and related drugs that have been of major benefit in treating Parkinson's disease, but if given in large doses they may cause nausea, faintness and weakness as additional side-effects.

Antirheumatic drugs
Mild antirheumatics include aspirin and similar preparations. Strong antirheumatic drugs include those based on phenylbutazone and indomethacin which are effective but often cause peptic ulcers and blood disorders. Occasionally injections of gold salts and other drugs are used. Pain-killing drugs are often used in combination with anti-rheumatic drugs in the treatment of arthritic disorders. In certain cases cortisone and other steroids may be required.

Antispasmodic drugs
These drugs relax smooth muscle in the intestine and the lungs. Intestinal antispasmodics can be given in the form of tablets or injections to relieve diarrhea or colic. Antispasmodics for the lungs are often called bronchodilators and can be given as tablets, or they can be inhaled. They are used particularly in the treatment of types of asthma.

Antiviral drugs
There are relatively few antiviral drugs. Some are used in the treatment of shingles, cold sores and virus infections of the eye. Research is currently in progress to develop antiviral drugs that may help to combat influenza and other virus infections.

Corticosteroid drugs
Corticosteroids are synthesized as cortisol or as chemical modifications of it to increase its effective strength. They prevent the body reacting to internal or external irritants and diseases by interfering with the body's normal reac-

tions to infection and by reducing inflammation. The drugs can be used in the form of eye and ear preparations; in nose drops and sprays, for the treatment of asthma; and in other different forms such as creams, to treat such skin conditions as eczema and psoriasis. Injections of corticosteroids are sometimes given directly into joints in certain forms of arthritis. Corticosteroid drugs taken by mouth will prevent the adrenal gland reacting to the stress of accidents, illnesses or surgery and this effect will persist for some months after the dosage of the drug has been stopped. Large amounts, taken over a long time, may cause a loss of calcium from the bones, an increase in weight, abnormal skin markings and a roundness in the shape of the face.

Cytotoxic drugs
These drugs destroy cancer cells and are used in the chemical treatment (chemotherapy) of cancer.

Diuretics
Diuretics increase the loss of water and salts through the kidneys. They are often used to treat heart diseases and some forms of kidney disease. Additional potassium salts should be given with some preparations if they are used for any length of time, to prevent muscle weakness.

Heart and blood-pressure drugs
Digoxin is used in heart failure and in some cases of tachycardia (rapid heartbeat) to increase the strength of the heart muscle and to reduce the pulse rate. Blood pressure can be reduced by a variety of drugs, including diuretics and the beta-adrenergic blocking agents that work by preventing the action of adrenalin.

Hormones
Adrenalin is used to treat severe allergic reactions (anaphylaxis) and severe asthma. It causes palpitations, sweating and a sense of anxiety. It may also be used as a heart stimulant. Thyroid hormone (thyroxine) is used in the treatment of hypothyroidism (myxoedema). Preparations from the pituitary gland, e.g. vasopressin, the antidiuretic hormone, are used to stimulate the contraction of blood vessels. Female sex hormones, such as estrogen, are used to treat menstrual disorders, in the contraceptive pill and in treating cancer of the prostate gland in men. Male hormones, known as androgens, and synthetic preparations are used to increase body strength after a debilitating illness.

Hypnotic and sedative drugs
These are used to treat insomnia. The barbiturate group are potentially addictive and may be fatal in overdosage. All these drugs tend to reduce dreaming and when they are stopped a period of one to two weeks of lighter sleep and of increased dreaming commonly occurs.

Laxatives
Laxatives stimulate bowel function. There are three main groups. Some act by increasing the bulk of the feces, either by adding insoluble salts or non-digestible vegetable fibre.

Others soften and lubricate feces. The third group stimulates bowel-wall contractions.

Pain-killing drugs

Mild pain-killers are based on aspirin and similar drugs. Occasionally they may cause skin rashes or intestinal bleeding, particularly if used to excess. Moderate pain-killers are based on codeine and similar chemicals. Their most common side-effect is constipation. Strong pain-killers such as morphine are derived from the opiate group. These drugs are sedative and addictive but are useful after operations and accidents or in the treatment of advanced cancer, when the relief of pain is more important than avoiding possible side-effects.

Tranquillizers

Minor hypnotics and sedatives used in small amounts act as tranquillizers. The benzodiazepines (Valium, Librium, etc.) are frequently used in the treatment of anxiety. They are also used with antidepressant drugs. They seldom cause adverse reactions apart from giving an artificial sense of elation and sometimes drowsiness. It is dangerous to drink alcohol when taking these drugs. Their most harmful side-effect is the sense of psychological dependence they may encourage. Major tranquillizers often have an antinausea and sedative effect. They are used in mental illnesses such as schizophrenia and alcoholism. Occasionally they cause liver damage.

Vaccines

Vaccines are used to create immunity and so are used to protect the body against infections. They are commonly made from a killed or weakened variety of the organism which causes the disease. Babies and children should be protected by vaccination against diphtheria, whooping cough, tetanus, poliomyelitis, measles, German measles (rubella) and tuberculosis. Many countries require injections with International Certificates of Vaccination against cholera and yellow fever to be given to travellers before they visit certain areas of the world where these diseases exist. Typhoid, typhus and plague vaccines are also available and may also be required by immigration authorities in some countries. Travellers should be vaccinated before they leave their home country. See A–Z: Immunization.

Vaso-constrictive drugs

These are used to cause blood vessels to contract. Adrenalin is sometimes used in cases of severe shock to raise the patient's blood pressure. Ergotamine is used in some anti-migraine preparations but it should only be taken at the onset of symptoms – excessive use may cause vomiting.

Vaso-dilator drugs

Vaso-dilators are used to expand blood vessels. They are used in angina pectoris to relieve or prevent heart pain and are usually prepared in a form that can be inhaled, chewed or swallowed. On exercise they may cause palpitations and flushing.

INDEX

For quick reference, index entries for the FIRST AID section are printed in red
Numerals in **bold** indicate a main entry.

A

Abdomen, burst, **19**
Abdominal pain, **19**, 37, 38, 43, 92,
  101, 105, 115, 116, 123, 124, 126,
  128, 129, 130, 132, 133, 136, 137,
  143, 146, 147, 152, 157, 162, 166,
  167
  see also Indigestion *and* Stomach
  ache
Abortion, **101–2**, 120, 141, 152
Abrasion, 7, **19**
Abscess, **102**, 104, 109, 127, 162,
  166
Accidents
  to children, 25, 30, 66–7
  domestic, **66–7**
  first aid at, 6, **11–18**
  hiking, 58
  ice, 27, **59–60**
  and the moving of victims, 11, 21,
  29–31, **38–9**, 121
  procedure at an accident, 10, **51–2**
  road, 6, **10**, 51–2
Achilles tendon, **102**
Acne, **102**
Adenoids, **102**, 113, 156, 160
A.I.D.S. (Acquired Immune
  Deficiency Syndrome), **102–3**,
  164
Air travel, fitness for, 27, 46
Airway, clearing the, 11, **13**, 15, 17
Alcohol, 53, 68, 124, 126, 131, 133,
  136, 139, 161, 162, 166, 168, 170,
  172
  and driving, 53, 184–5
Alcoholism, 44, **103**, 115, 121, 130,
  133, 138, 150, 172
Allergic rhinitis *see* Hay fever
Allergy, **19–20**, 22, 40, 42, 43, **103**,
  104, 113, 117, 121, 125, 131, 135,
  137, 143, 151, 152, 155, 166, 168,
  169, 171
Altitude sickness, **103**
Amebic dysentery *see* Dysentery
Amenorrhea *see* Menstrual
  disorders
Amputation, accidental, **19**
Anal problems, **104**, 127
  abscess, 103
  bleeding, 22, 92, 93, 104, 116, 117,
  123, 137
  fissure-in-ano, 104, 117
  hemorrhoids, **36**, 104, **131–2**, 137,
  149
  itching, 37, 104, 137
  lump, 37, 104, 133
Anaphylaxis, 20, 103, **104**
Anatomy and physiology, **81–90**
Anemia, 69, **104**, 111, 112, 118, 126,
  136, 137, 138, 139, 145, 148, 165
Angina pectoris, 36, **104–5**, 114,
  134, 172
Animal bites, 21, 150, 167
Ankylosing spondylitis *see*
  Spondylitis and spondylosis

Ankylosis, **105**
Anorexia nervosa, **105**, 141, 166
Anxiety, 103, **105**, 106, 107, 109,
  110, 111, 114, 121, 122, 124, 126,
  128, 130, 132, 134, 136, 137, 140,
  142, 143, 144, 145, 149, 151, 153,
  163, 164, 169, 171, 172
Appendicitis, 101, **105**, 116, 147, 151
Arm injuries, bandaging, 34–5, **42**
Arteries, 86
  see also Angina pectoris,
  Arteriosclerosis, Embolus *and*
  Thrombosis
Arteriosclerosis, 74, **105–6**, 109,
  112, 115, 119, 122, 129, 144, 156,
  158, 159
Arthritis, 46, 75, 105, **106**, 111, 131,
  132, 144, 153, 157, 158, 166, 170,
  171
Artificial respiration, 11, **13–17**
Asbestosis *see* Pneumoconiosis
Asphyxiation, **20**
  see also Choking
Asthma, **20**, 22, 46, **106**, 111, 114,
  125, 131, 147, 169, 170, 171
Astigmatism, **106**
Athlete's foot, **106**, 160, 169
Autism, **106**

B

Babies *see* Infants
Bacillary dysentery *see* Dysentery
Backache, 38, 97, 101, **106–7**, 126,
  137, 139, 142, 143, 146, 149, 150,
  153, 157, 163
  what to do, **98**
  see also Slipped disc *and* Spine
Back injuries, **20–1**, 107
  see also Slipped disc *and* Spine
Bad breath, **107**
Balance, 85, 143
Balanitis *see* Foreskin, sore
Bandaging *see* Fractures, bandaging
Basal cell carcinoma *see* Rodent
  ulcer
Bat ear, **107**
B.C.G. vaccine *see* Tuberculosis,
  immunization
Bed bath, 72–3, 75
Bedsore, **107**
Bedwetting, **107**, 136
Bell's palsy, **107**
Bent or curved back, **107–8**, 134,
  144, 147
Bicycling safety, 53, 54, **55**
Birth control, 102
  see also Contraception
Birthmark, **108**
Bites, **21**
  see also Animal bites, Insect bites
  and stings *and* Snakebite
Black eye, 28
Blackhead *see* Acne
Bladder, 81, 89, 127, 149, 156, 163
  bleeding from the, 22

inflammation of the, 119
  see also Cystitis *and*
  Incontinence
Blanket supports, 73
Bleeding, 11, 19, **21–2**, 30, 42, 103,
  104, 108, 115, 126, 170
  anal, 22, 92, 93, 104, 116, 117,
  123, 137
  from the bladder, 22
  after childbirth, 25
  from the ear, 22, 27
  intestinal, 172
  from the mouth, 22
  from the nose, 39, 103, **144**, 167
  ulcer, 162
  vaginal, 38, 112, 141, 142, **163–4**
Blindness, **108**, 113, 122, 130, 142,
  156
Blister, 22, 42, **108**, 116, 121, 135,
  155
Blood, 81, 86
  spitting of, 96, **108**
  in the stools, 122, 124
  in urine, 99, 112, 119, 137, 143,
  149, 157, **163,**
  in vomit, 44
  see also Bleeding, Circulation
  and Leukemia
Blood pressure, 74, 104, 105, **108–9,**
  117, 119, 126, 132, 148, 157, 171,
  172
Blue baby, **109**, 115
Boating safety, 60–1, 63–4
Body odour, **109**
Boil *see* Abscess
Bones, 81, 82–3, 144, 161
  see also Fractures
Botulism, 128
Bow-legs, **109**, 138, 151
Bradycardia *see* Palpitations
Brain, 81, 84
  infections, 125, 140
  see also Concussion,
  Encephalitis, Hydrocephalus,
  Meningitis *and* Stroke
Breast examination, **109**, 112, 162
Breast problems, **109–10**, 117
  abscess, 109
  babies' breasts, 109–10
  development, 110
  inflammation, 142, 148
  lump, 110, 162
  mastitis, 110
  nipple disease, 110
  size, 110
  tenderness, 110, 149
Breath-holding attack, **110–11**
Breathing
  checking for, 6, 11, **12**, 18
  problems, 22, 95, 96, 103, 104,
  111, 119, 125, 132, 144, 148
  see also Asthma, Bronchitis,
  Emphysema, Lungs, Pleurisy,
  Pneumonia, Respiratory system,
  Tracheitis *and* Tuberculosis
Breathlessness *see* Breathing
  problems
Bromhidrosis *see* Body odour
Bronchitis, 74, 106, 108, **111,** 118,
  125, 136, 140, 147, 156, 161
Bruising, 22, 162
Bunion, 75, **111**
Burns, 11, 22, **23**, 28, 152

Bursitis, **111–12,** 129, 158

C

Calf pain on walking, 105, **112,**
  119
Camping, **55–7**
Cancer, 103, 108, 110, 111, **112–13,**
  117, 119, 125, 129, 133, 138, 140,
  141, 147, 148, 149, 156, 162, 171,
  172
Candidiasis *see* Moniliasis
Canoeing safety, 61
Capsulitis, 112, **113,** 129, 158
Carbuncle *see* Abscess
Cardio-pulmonary resuscitation,
  11, **16**
Carpal tunnel syndrome, **113**
Cartilage, torn, **113,** 166
Car travel, 46–7
  fitness to drive, 52–3, 126,
  168
  insurance, 10, 50, 51
  safety, 9, 49–53
  towing trailers, 55–7
  see also Country-by-country
  medical and motoring
  requirements, Road accidents
  and Travel, sickness
Cataract, 74, 108, **113,** 130
Catarrh, 102, **113,** 116, 118, 120,
  140, 144, 145, 148, 155, 156, 166,
  167
Chancre, **114,** 158
Chancroid, **114,** 164
Charts of what to do *see* Symptoms:
  Charts of what to do
Checklists
  action at a road crash, 10, 51–2
  backpack survival kit, 59
  car safety, 49–50
  domestic accident prevention, 66
  drugs for the home, 6, 7
  drugs for travelling abroad, 48
  first aid at an accident, 11
  first aid cabinet, 7
  first aid kit, 8–9
  household aids for the elderly, 75
  immunizations for travellers, 47
  insurance claim, 52
Chemical
  burns, 23
  poisoning, 148
Chemicals in the eye, 28
Chest
  injuries, 30
  pain, 96, 107, **114,** 132, 147,
  161
  pain, what to do, **95**
  tightness, **114**
  see also Heart, Lungs *and*
  Respiratory system
Chickenpox, 22, 40, **114,** 125, 133,
  151, 155
Chilblain, **114,** 115, 120, 151
Childbirth, **114–15,** 126, 147, 148,
  149
  emergency, 23–5
  stillbirth, 156, **157**
Children
  accidents to, 25, 41, 66
  in cars, 49

choking, 18
mouth-to-mouth resuscitation of, 15
and safe storage of medicines, 6, 66–7
see also Infants
Chloasma, **115**
Choking, 11, 17
Cholecystitis *see* Gall-bladder, disorders
Cholera, **115,** 122
immunization, 47, 115, 134, 172, 184–5
Cholesterol, 68, 69, 105, 129, 132
Circulation, 68, 81, 86, 129
problems, **115**
see also Bleeding, Blood, Embolus, Heart *and* Thrombosis
Circumcision, **115,** 128
Cirrhosis, 103, 112, **115,** 117, 137, 138, 165
Clearing the airway, 11, **13,** 15, 17
Coitus interruptus, 117
Cold, common, 7, 27, 46, 74, 106, 108, 111, 113, **115–16,** 117, 118, 144, 145, 147, 155, 163, 166
Cold compress *see* Ice pack
Cold sore, **116,** 133, 170
Colic, 101, **116,** 119, 123, 129, 137, 157, 166, 167, 170
Colitis, 101, 103, 112, **116,** 122, 127, 137
Colon, 46, 116
Collarbone, fractured, 30
Coma *see* Unconsciousness
Concussion, 25, 36, **116**
Condom, 117
Conjunctivitis, **116–17,** 126, 131, 137, 140, 158
Consciousness, maintaining, 18
Constipation, 7, 75, 92, 104, 107, 116, **117,** 133, 136, 137, 149, 162, 169, 171–2
what to do, **92**
Contraception, **117–18,** 163
contraceptive pill, 110, 115, 117–18, 141, 143, 146, 159, 163, 164, 166, 171
foams, creams and gels, 117, 118
IUCD (IUD), 118, 163
'rhythm method,' 118
sterilization, 117, 118
vasectomy, 117
Convulsions and fits, 11, **25–6,** 44, 103, **118,** 124, 126, 127, 135, 141
Corn, 75, **118**
Coronary thrombosis *see* Heart attack
Cough, 7, 95, 107, 111, 112, **118–19,** 125, 132, 136, 140, 147, 161, 162, 166, 167
what to do, **96**
Crabs *see* Lice
Cramp, 26, 43, **119,** 146
Cretinism, 160
Croup, 111, **119**
Crying, infant, **119**
Curved back *see* Bent or curved back
Cyst, sebaceous, 110, **119**
Cystitis, 44, **119–20,** 131, 150, 163

D

D and C (Dilatation and curettage), 102, **120,** 141, 146
Dead fingers, 115, **120**
Deafness, 74, 94, 102, **120,** 130, 140, 142, 145, 166
what to do, **96**
Death, what to do, **120–1**
Dehydration, 26, 29, 44, 93, 115, 117, 123, 161, 163, 166, 167
Delirium, 94, **121,** 124, 127, 139, 162
Delirium tremens, 103, **121,** 124
Dental problems, 26, 107, 130
see also Mouth, Teeth, Teething *and* Toothache
Depression, 105, 118, **121,** 124, 130, 132, 134, 136, 139, 140, 141, 143, 144, 149, 153
Dermatitis, 120, **121,** 137, 144, 151, 171
see also specific skin disorders
Detached retina, 108, **121–2**
Diabetes, 44, 46, 74, 105, 108, 117, **122,** 137, 144, 148, 153, 163, 164, 169
emergencies, 27, 122
Diaper rash, 40, **122,** 128
Diaphragm, hiatus hernia of the, **133–4**
Diaphragm (Dutch cap), 117, 118
Diarrhea, 7, 26, 29, 59, 92, 93, 101, 103, 115, 116, 119, **122,** 123, 124, 128, 129, 132, 137, 160, 166, 167, 169, 170
in babies, **122**
traveller's diarrhea, 48, 122, **161,** 169
what to do, **93**
Diet, 45, **68–70,** 70, 72, 75, 102, 104, 105, 107, 112, 115, 116, 117, 119, 122, 123, 125, 126, 130, 132, 133, 136, 137, 139, 143, 144, 148, 151, 155, 161, 162, 166, 167
see also Cholesterol, Iron *and* Vitamins
Digestive system, 68, 81, 88, 129
see also Colitis, Constipation, Diarrhea, Diverticulitis, Dysentery, Flatulence, Gastritis, Indigestion, Polyp, Typhoid *and* Wind
Dilatation and curettage *see* D and C
Diphtheria, **123,** 148, 156
immunization, 134, 135, 172
Disabled people, travel abroad, 184–5
Dislocations, 27, **123**
Disposal of medicines, 6
Diverticulitis, 103, 116, 122, **123,** 137, 147
Dizziness
what to do, **91**
Domestic accidents *see* Accidents, domestic
Dressings, 7, 8, 33, 59
Driving
and alcohol, 53, 184–5
and drugs, 53, 168, 170
fitness to drive, **52–3,** 126, 168
see also Car travel, Country-by-country medical and motoring requirements *and* Road accidents

Drowning, **27**
Drug abuse, 44, 68, 102, 121, **123–4,**
133, 150, 153
  cannabis, 124
  depressants, 123
  opiates, 123–4
  psychedelics, 124
  stimulants, 123
Drugs, 53, **168–72**
  anesthetics, 133, **168**
  antacids, 130, 134, 136, 143, 162,
  168
  antiallergic, 20, **168**
  antibiotics, 21, 48, 65, 102, 103,
  109, 110, 111, 114, 115, 120, 123,
  124, 128, 129, 131, 133, 135, 136,
  140, 141, 143, 144, 145, 147, 149,
  150, 151, 152, 155, 158, 159, 161,
  162, 164, 167, **168,** 169
  anticoagulants, 132, 159, **168–9**
  anticonvulsants, **169**
  antidepressants, 105, 121, **169,**
  172
  antidiabetic, 122, **169**
  antidiarrheal, 116, 122, 128, 161,
  169
  antiepileptic, 126
  antifungal, 106, 122, 142, 160,
  167, **169**
  antihistamines, 20, 37, 48, 59,
  102, 103, 104, 106, 113, 114, 116,
  119, 125, 132, 137, 143, 145, 155,
  168, **169–70**
  anti-inflammatory, 147, 171
  antimalarial, **170**
  antinausea and antiemetic, 43, 46,
  48, 141, 142, 143, 161, **170,** 172
  anti-Parkinsonian, 146, **170**
  antirheumatic, 106, 113, 129, 131,
  153, 156, 157, 158, 159, 162, 166,
  170
  antispasmodic, 116, 120, 123,
  137, 157, 169, **170**
  antiviral, 116, 133, 155, **170**
  appetite-depressant, 144
  bronchodilators, 106, 170
  checklist, 7
  corticosteroid, 103, 104, 106, 107,
  113, 125, 129, 142, 158, 159, 162,
  164, 168, **170–1**
  cytotoxic, 112, 138, 140, 150, **171**
  and discoloration of urine, 163
  disposal of, 6
  diuretics, 103, 132, 149, **171**
  and driving, 53, 168, 170
  heart and blood pressure, 104,
  109, 112, 124, 132, **171**
  hormones, 117, 144, **171**
  hypnotic and sedative, 46, 75,
  105, 111, 121, 123, 124, 126, 139,
  147, 167, 168, 169, **171,** 172
  laxative, 75, 117, 122, 133, **171–2**
  pain-killing, 170, **172**
  reactions to, 20, 92, 104, 130, 132,
  143, 160, 162, 164, 165, 166,
  168–72
  sedative *see* hypnotic and
  sedative *above*
  storage of, 6, 72
  tranquillizers, 105, 153, 168, 169,
  170, **172**
  for travelling abroad, 9, **48,** 122
  vaccines, 133, **172** (*see also*

Immunization)
  vaso-constrictive, **172**
  vaso-dilator, **172**
  see also Contraception,
  contraceptive pill
Dumbness, 120
Dysentery, 122, **124,** 133
Dysmenorrhea *see* Periods,
painful
Dyspepsia *see* Indigestion

E

Ear
  bat ear, **107**
  bleeding from the, 22, 27
  burst eardrum, 27, 125, 145
  discharge from the, 94, 120, **125,**
  145
  drops, 120, 125, 145
  foreign body in the, 27, 120
  infections, 102, 120, 132, 143, 171
  injuries, **27**
  structure, 81, 85
  wax, 120, 145, **166–7**
  see also Deafness, Mastoiditis,
  Ménière's disease, Otitis externa
  and Otitis media
Earache, 120, **125,** 145, 166
  what to do, **94**
Eczema, 106, 121, 122, **125,** 135,
137, 144, 164, 171
Electrical
  burns, 23, **28**
  safety, 66–7
Electric shock, **28**
Embolus, 108, 111, **125,** 129, 147,
158, 159
Emphysema, 106, 111, **125,** 147
Encephalitis, 121, **125,** 132, 133,
140, 141, 146, 167
Endocrine system, 81, 90
Enteric fever *see* Typhoid
Epilepsy, 44, 46, 52, 111, 117, 118,
125–6, 169
Epistaxis *see* Nosebleed
Exercise, 45, 53, 68, 70–1, 75, 102,
104, 105, 106, 112, 115, 125, 127,
132, 145, 148
Exhibitionism, 154
Exposure *see* Hypothermia
Eye
  black eye, **28**
  chemicals in the, **28**
  drops, 74, 168
  foreign body in the, **28**
  gritty feeling in the, **131**
  infections, 170, 171
  injuries, **28**
  sore or red eye, 116, 126, 130
  sore or red eye, what to do, **100**
  structure, 81, 85
  see also Astigmatism, Blindness,
  Cataract, Conjunctivitis,
  Detached retina, Farsightedness,
  Glaucoma, Iritis, Migraine *and*
  Nearsightedness
Eyelids
  sore and swollen, **100,** 117, **126,**
  143
  stys, **43,** 126, 158
  twitching, **126**

F

Facial fractures, 30
Fainting, 18, 36, 91, 104, 108, 109,
　115, 118, 125, **126**, 170
　see also Unconsciousness
False pains (in pregnancy), **126**
Farsightedness, 74, **126,**
Fatigue *see* Malaise
Fetishism, 154
Fever, 7, 25, 26, 27, **29**, 40, 46, 72, 92,
　94, 95, 96, 97, 98, 99, 100, 101,
　103, 105, 107, 111, 114, 115, 116,
　119, 121, 123, 124, 125, **126–7**,
　128, 130, 132, 133, 136, 138, 139,
　140, 142, 143, 145, 147, 150, 151,
　152, 155, 156, 157, 158, 159, 160,
　161, 162, 163, 166, 167
　what to do, **94**
Fever sore *see* Cold sore
Fibroid, **127**, 129, 163
Fibrositis, **127**, 128, 157
Finger
　hair round a, **36**
　ring stuck on a, **41**
Fingers, dead, 115, **120**
First aid
　at accidents, 6, 10, **11–18**
　equipment, 6, 7, **8–9**, 48, 49, 50,
　59, 65
Fishhook injuries, **29**
Fissure-in-ano, 104, 117
Fistula, 103, **127**
Fitness
　to drive, **52–3**, 126
　to travel, 27, **46–7**, 145
Fits *see* Convulsions and fits
Flat foot, **127**
Flatulence, **128**, 136, 157
Flooding, vaginal, **128**
'Flu *see* Influenza
Food
　chemical substances in, 112
　poisoning, **29**, 48, 56, 64, 124,
　128, 130, 161, 162, 165
　see also Diet
Foot
　athlete's foot, **106**, 160, 169
　bandaging the, 32
　care for the elderly, 75
　disorders, 106, 111, 118, 127, 160,
　164–5
　injuries, **29**, 42, 108, 129
Foreskin, sore, 115, **128**
Fractures, 11, 21, **29–35**, 39, 40, 42,
　107, 120, **128**, 144, 157
　bandaging, **30–5**
Frigidity, 153, 154
Frostbite, **35**, 114, 129
Frozen shoulder, 113, **129**
Frustration, sexual *see* Sex
　problems *and* Sexuality
Furuncle *see* Abscess

G

Gall-bladder, 88
　disorders, 116, 128, **129**, 136, 137,
　138
Gangrene, 122, 125, **129**, 159
Gastric 'flu, 101, 116, 122, 128, **129**,
　130, 165

Gastritis, 103, **130**, 136, 143, 157
Genu valgum *see* Knock-knee
Genu varum *see* Bow-legs
German measles, 40, 113, 120, **130**
　immunization, 134, 172
Gingivitis, 107, 108, **130**, 156
Glands
　adrenal, 90, 115, 171
　endocrine, 68, 81, 90, 144
　lymph, 68, 102, 103, 114, 136, 139
　pancreas, 90, 122
　parathyroid, 90
　parotid, 142
　pituitary, 90, 122, 171
　prostate, 44, 75, 135–6, 149, 163,
　171
　thyroid, 90, 144, 145, 160, 171
Glandular fever *see* Infectious
　mononucleosis
Glaucoma, 108, **130**
Glossitis, **130–1**
Glue-sniffing, 124
Gonorrhea, **131**, 144, 146, 149, 164
Gout, **131**, 157
Granuloma inguinale, **131**, 164
Grazes *see* Abrasion
Gripe *see* Colic
Gritty feeling in the eye, **131**
Gumboil, 26, 107, 130, **131**, 161
Gunshot wounds, **35**

H

Hair round a finger, **36**
Halitosis *see* Bad breath
Hang gliding, 46
Hardening of the arteries *see*
　Arteriosclerosis
Hay fever, 106, 125, **131**, 137, 148
Headache, 7, 96, 97, 103, 116, 121,
　125, 127, 128, **132**, 136, 140, 141,
　142, 147, 149, 157, 158, 162, 165
　what to do, **97**
　see also Migraine
Head injuries, 25, 27, 30, 33, **36**, 44,
　116, 132
　bandaging, 33, 26
Health
　and fitness, **68–71**
　insurance, 48, 50, 184–5
　on vacation, 9, **45–65**, 66, 161
Heart
　attack, **36**, 42, 46, 68, 74, 104,
　105, 109, 111, 129, **132**, 156,
　159
　beat, 6, 12
　and circulation, 81, 86
　disorders, 46, 70, 104, 130, 144,
　145, 171
　failure, 111, 115, 118, 123, **132**,
　165, 171
　massage, 12, **13–14**, 16, 17
　see also Blue baby, Pulse *and*
　Rheumatic fever
Heartburn, **132–3**, 134, 136, 162
Heat exhaustion, 29, **36**, 43
Heatstroke, 29, **37**
Heberden's nodes, **132**
Heimlich maneuver, 17–18
Hematuria *see* Urine, blood in
Hemoptysis *see* Blood, spitting of
Hemorrhage *see* Bleeding

Hemorrhoids, 37, 104, **133**, 137, 149
Hepatitis, 115, 124, **133**, 137, 138, 166
  immunization, 47, 133, 134, 135, 184–5
Hernia *see* Hiatus hernia *and* Rupture
Herpes, 114, **133**, 136, 155
  genitalis, **133**, 164, 166
  simplex, 116, 133
  zoster *see* Shingles
Hiatus hernia, 128, **133–4**, 136, 152
Hiccups, 37, **134**, 136
Hiking, **58–9**
Hole-in-the-heart baby, 109, 115
Holger-Nielsen method of artificial respiration, 13, 16–17, 40
Homosexuality, 102–3, 154
Hormones, 81, 90, 109, 117, 122, 128, 141, 144, 153, 160, **171**
Housemaid's knee, 112
Hunchback, **134**
Hydrocephalus, 157
Hydrophobia *see* Rabies
Hygiene
  camping, 56
  personal, 102, 109, 115, 135, 138, 146, 162
  see also Food poisoning *and* Water contamination
Hyperglycemic coma, 27, 122
Hypermetropia *see* Long-sightedness
Hypertension *see* Blood pressure
Hyperthyroidism *see* Thyroid problems
Hyperuricemia *see* Gout
Hypochondria, **134**
Hypoglycemic coma, 27, 122, 169
Hypotension *see* Blood pressure
Hypothermia, 37, 58, 60, 62, 75
Hypothyroidism *see* Thyroid problems
Hysteria, **134**, 143, 145

I

Ice accidents, 27, **59–60**
Ice pack (cold compress), 37
Immunization, **47, 134–5**, 172, 184–5
  cholera, 47, 115, 172, 184–5
  diphtheria, 134, 172
  German measles, 134, 172
  hepatitis, 47, 133, 135, 184–5
  influenza, 135
  malaria, 184–5
  measles, 135, 172
  mumps, 135, **142**
  plague, 172
  poliomyelitis, 47, 135, 148, 172, 184–5
  rabies, 21, 135
  temporary, 135
  tetanus, 19, 21, 22, 29, 42, 47, 134, 135, **159**, 172
  for the traveller, **47, 134–5**, 172, 184–5
  tuberculosis, 135, 172

typhoid, 47, 135, 172, 184–5
typhus, 47, 135, 172
whooping cough, 134, 135, 172
yellow fever, 47, 135, 167, 172
Impetigo, 122, **135,**
Impotence, 153
Incest, 154
Incontinence, 75, 99, 104, 126, **135–6,** 149
Indigestion, 7, 19, 114, 127, 132–3, **136,** 157, 163
  see also Abdominal pain *and* Stomach ache
Infants
  babies' breasts, 109–10
  checklist for home medicine cabinet, 7
  crying, **119**
  heart massage of, 14
  mouth-to-mouth/nose resuscitation of, 15
  newborn, 24–5
Infectious illnesses *see specific diseases*
Infectious mononucleosis, 133, **136,** 156
Influenza, 74, **136,** 156, 170
  immunization, 135
Ingrowing toenail, **160**
Insect bites and stings, 20, 22, **37–8,** 104, 143, 167, 169
Insomnia, 105, 121, 124, 125, **136,** 167, 171
Insulin *see* Drugs, antidiabetic
Insurance
  motor, 10, 50, 51
  travel, 48, 50, 184–5
Intermittent claudication *see* Calf pain on walking
Internal injuries, 22, 35
Intussusception, 103, 104, 116, **137**
Iritis, **137**
Iron, 69, 104, 148
Irritable bowel syndrome, 116, **137**
Itching, 40, 42, **137**
  anal, 36, 104, 137
  vulval, 137, 164
  see also Athlete's foot, Chilblain, Conjunctivitis, Eczema, German measles, Hemorrhoids, Lice, Nettle rash, Otitis externa, Rash, Scabies *and* Shingles
IUCD (IUD) (Intra-Uterine Contraceptive Device), 98, 99, 118

J

Jaundice, 129, 133, 136, **137,** 138, 163, 167
Jaw, fractured, 30
Jellyfish stings, 43, 143
Jet lag, 46
Jogging, 70
Joints, 81, 82–3
  painful, 106
  painful, what to do, **97**
  see also Ankylosis, Arthritis, Bursitis, Capsulitis, Dislocations, Gout *and* Rheumatic fever

K

Kidneys, 81, 89
  disorders of the, 101, 106, 109,
  116, 119, 122, 131, 134, **137**, 139,
  150, 163, 165, 171
  see also Nephritis,
  Pyelonephritis, Stone in kidney,
  Urination *and* Urine
Kiss-of-life *see* Mouth-to-mouth
  resuscitation
Knock-knee, 109, **138**, 151

L

Labour *see* Childbirth
Laryngitis, **138**, 161
Law and accident procedures, 10,
  51–2
Leg injuries, bandaging, 32, 33,
  42
Lesbianism, 154
Leukemia, 112, **138**
Lice, **138**, 162, 164
'Lightening' (in pregnancy), **138**,
  148
Lightning injuries, 64
Listlessness *see* Malaise
Liver disorders, 103, 115, 117, 124,
  138, 165, 172
  see also Cirrhosis *and* Hepatitis
Lockjaw *see* Tetanus
Lumbago *see* Backache
Lump *see* Tumour
Lungs, 81, 87
  disorders of the, 46, 70, 103, 107,
  108, 148, 156
  see also Respiratory system
Lymphatic system, 68, 102, 103,
  112, 114, 136, 139
Lymphogranuloma venereum, **139**,
  164

M

Malaise, 111, 112, 116, 127, 136,
  138, **139**, 140, 155, 160, 161
Malaria, 48, 104, **139**, 170
  immunization, 184–5
Mania, 121, **139**, 153
Manic-depressive illness, 121, **139**
Masochism, 154
Mastitis, 110
Mastoiditis, 125, **139**, 145
Masturbation, **140**, 153, 154
Measles, 40, 117, 125, **140**, 151, 155
  immunization, 135, 172
Medical
  advice, 91, 101, 184–5
  check-ups, 46
  words, **76–80**
Medicines, 6–9
  disposal of, 6
  storage of, 6, 66–7
  see also Drugs
Meditation, 71
Melanoma, 112, **140**
Ménière's disease, **140**
Meningitis, 118, 132, **141**, 157
Menopause, 112, 128, **141**, 146, 149,
  163, 164

Menstrual disorders, 120, **141**, 144,
  160, 163, 171
  amenorrhea, 105, 141
  nipple secretion, 110
  premenstrual tension, 113, **148–9**
Menstruation *see* Periods
Migraine, 38, 108, 132, **141**, 143,
  161, 166, 172
Miscarriage, 38, 102, 128, **141–2**,
  152, 156, 163
Moles, 108, 112
Moniliasis, 122, **142**, 164, 167, 169
Mononucleosis, infectious *see*
  Infectious mononucleosis
Morning sickness, **142**, 143, 148
Motion sickness *see* Travel
  sickness
Motorcycling
  accidents, 10, 53
  safety, **53–5**
Motoring requirements, country-by-
  country, 184–5
Mountain climbing, 46
Mountain sickness *see* Altitude
  sickness
Mouth
  bleeding from the, 22
  care, 73, 75
  infections, 107, 108
  injuries, 13, 15, 16, **38**, 40
  obstructions, 13
  ulcer, 26, **163**
  see also Dental problems,
  Gingivitis, Glossitis, Gumboil,
  Moniliasis, Teeth, Teething *and*
  Toothache
Mouth-to-mouth resuscitation, 11,
  13, **15**, 16
Mouth-to-nose resuscitation, **15**,
  16
Moving the patient, 11, 21, **29–31**,
  38–9, 58, 121
Mucous colitis *see* Irritable bowel
  syndrome
Multiple sclerosis, 108, **142**
Mumps, 120, **142**, 148
  immunization, 135
Muscles, 81, 82–3, 107, 119, 126,
  157
  pulled, **40**, 107, 112
  see also Paralysis
Myocardial infarction *see* Heart
  attack
Myxedema *see* Thyroid problems

N

Narcissism, 154
Nausea, 96, 101, 103, 105, 118, 124,
  126, 130, 132, 133, 136, 140, 141,
  143, 157, 162, 166, 170
Nearsightedness, **143**
Neck
  fractured, 29
  stiff, 127, 132, 140, 147, **157**
Nephritis, **143**, 151, 152, 158, 163
Nervous system, 81, 84
  disorders of the, 46, 68, 108, 118,
  123, 136, 141, 146, 153, 158, 161
  see also Multiple sclerosis,
  Neuralgia, Paralysis, Parkinson's

disease, Polyneuritis *and* Shingles
Nettle rash (urticaria), 125, 137, **143**
Neuralgia, 132
Neurosis, **143**, 144
Night
blindness, 165
sweats, **143**
terrors, **143–4**
Nipple disease *see* Breast problems
Nits *see* Lice
Nocturnal enuresis *see* Bedwetting
Nonspecific urethritis (NSU), 131, **144**, 146, 164
Nose
drops, 73, 102, 113, 120, 145, 155, 171
infections, 107, 156
injuries, 16, **39**, 123
mouth-to-nose resuscitation, 15, 16
structure, 81, 85
see also Catarrh, Hay fever *and* Sinusitis
Nosebleed, **39**, 104, **144**, 167

O

Obesity, 68, 69, 70, 74–5, 105, 109, 122, 134, **144**
Obsession, 143, **144**
Old age
care of the elderly, 45, 71, 75
household aids, 75
problems of, 45, 46–7, 52, **74–5**, 104, 108, 113, 115, 120, 122, 123, 132, 135–6, 144, 146, 147, 149, 160
Osteoarthritis *see* Arthritis
Osteomalacia *see* Rickets
Osteoporosis, 108, **144**
Otitis externa, 120, 125, **144–5**
Otitis media, 102, 120, 125, 132, 136, 139, 140, **145**, 166, 167
Otosclerosis *see* Deafness

P

Pain, abdominal *see* Abdominal pain
Paleness (pallor), 104, **145**
Palpitations, 103, 105, 121, 123, 141, **145**, 160, 171, 172
Papanicolaou smear *see* Smear test
Paralysis, 31, 52, 107, 127, 142, **145**, 148, 150, 153, 157, 158
Paranoia, 123, **145**, 152
Paratyphoid, 128
Parkinson's disease, 125, **146**, 170
Pedophilia, 155
Penis
discharge from the, 131, 144, **146**
inflammation of the, 153
zip-fastener injuries, 44
see also Circumcision *and* Foreskin, sore
Periods, 117, 118, 141, 144, **146**, 150, 163, 164
heavy, 69, 104, 118, 127–8
heavy, what to do, **99**

painful, 101, 107, 118, **146**
painful, what to do, **98**
see also Menstrual disorders
Peritonitis, **146–7**, 152, 162
Pertussis *see* Whooping cough
Pharynx, 85
Phlebitis, 115, **147**, 159
Physical problems with sex *see* Sex problems
Physiology *see* Anatomy and physiology
Piles *see* Hemorrhoids
Pink eye *see* Conjunctivitis
Pleurisy, 107, **147**
Pneumoconiosis, 111, **147**
Pneumonia, 74, 106, 111, 114, 118, 136, **147**, 167
Poisoning, 11, **40**, 44, 118, 148
see also Food poisoning *and* Water contamination
Poker back, **147**, 157
Poliomyelitis, 127, 145, **147–8**
immunization, 47, 135, 148, 172, 184–5
Polyneuritis, 103, 108, 123, 145, **148**, 165
Polyp, 104, 113, **148**, 162
Pregnancy, 98, 99, 110, 113, 114–15, 117, 118, 120, 122, 126, 127, 130, 134, 141, **148**, 150, 157, 163, 164, 166, 170
and air travel, 46
false pains, **126**
'lightening,' **138**, 148
miscarriage, 38, 102, 128, **141–2**, 152, 156, 163
morning sickness, **142**, 143, 148
quickening, 148, **150**
test, 141, **148**
see also Abortion, Childbirth, Contraception *and* Stillbirth
Premenstrual tension, 113, 146, **148–9**
Pressure sore *see* Bed sore
Prolapse
of the rectum, 104, **149**
of the womb, 75, 135, **149**, 163
Prostate problems, 44, 75, 135–6, **149**, 163, 171
Pruritus *see* Itching
Psoriasis, **149–50**, 171
Psychological problems with sex *see* Sex problems
Psychosis, 124, **150**, 152, 153
Puberty, 110, 144, **150**, 154
Pulled muscle, **40**
Pulse, checking the, 11, **12**, 18
Pulse rate, 145
see also Palpitations
Pyelonephritis, 107, 109, 119, **150**, 163

Q

Quickening, 148, **150**

R

Rabies, 21, **150**
immunization, 21, 135, 150
Rash, 7, 20, **40**, 42, 94, 125, 130, 140,

142–3, **151,** 152, 155, 158, 172
what to do, **100**
Raynaud's phenomenon, 114, 120,
151
Recovery position, 11, **18**
Rectum
polyp of the, 104
prolapse of the, 104, **149**
Relaxation, 68, 71
Reproductive system, 81, 90
Rescue from a height, **41**
Respiratory system, 81, 87
disorders and infections, 108,
109, 114, 115, 117, 122–3, 146,
147, 156
see also Asthma, Breathing,
Bronchitis, Cough, Croup,
Diaphragm, Emphysema, Lungs,
Pleurisy, Pneumonia, Tracheitis
and Tuberculosis
Resuscitation *see* Artificial
respiration
Retention of urine, **44,** 149, **163**
Retina, detached, 108, **121–2**
Rheumatic fever, **151,** 152, 158
Rheumatism, 108, 127, 147, **151,**
157, 170
Rheumatoid arthritis *see* Arthritis
Rhinitis, 155
allergic *see* Hay fever
vascomotor, 113
'Rhythm method', 118
Rib, fractured, 30
Rickets, 109, 144, **151,** 165
Ring stuck on a finger, **41**
Ringworm *see* Tinea
Road accidents, 6, **10,** 51–2
see also Safety, road
Rodent ulcer, 112, **151**
Rubella *see* German measles
Rubeola *see* Measles
Rupture (hernia), **37,** 111, 116, 147,
151–2
see also Hiatus hernia

S

Sadism, 154
Safety
and health, 45
in the home, 66–7
road, 9, 49–55, 184–5
Sailing, 60
Salmonella *see* Food poisoning *and*
Typhoid
Salpingitis, 128, 147, **152**
Scabies, 137, **152,** 164
Scalds, 23
Scarlet fever, 40, 117, 143, 151, **152,**
158
Scars, 102, 151, **152**
Schizophrenia, 150, **152–3,** 172
Sciatica, **153,** 155
Scrapes *see* Abrasion
Scratches *see* Abrasion
Scuba diving, 46, 61
Sea travel, 46
see also Travel, sickness
Seat belts, 49, 50, 184–5
Sebaceous cyst, 110, **119**
Sedation of infants, 7

Seizures *see* Convulsions and fits
Senses, 81, 85, 125
Sex problems, **153–4**
Sexuality, 139–40, 150, 153, **154–5**
Sexually transmitted diseases *see*
Venereal diseases
Sheath (condom), 117
Shingles, 22, 114, 133, **155,** 170
Shock, 18, 22, 23, 25, 27, 28, 30, 35,
41, 42, 44, 58, 104, 115, 132, 145,
172
Shoulder, frozen, 113, **128**
Sickroom, 45, **71–4**
Silicosis *see* Pneumoconiosis
Silvester method of artificial
respiration, 13, 16, **17**
Sinusitis, 27, 46, 113, 118, 132, 136,
140, **155,** 167
Skating, 59–60
Skiing, 59
Skin disorders *see* Dermatitis
Skull, fractured, 30
Sky diving, 46
Sleep-walking, **155**
Slings, 30, 35
Slipped disc, 153, **155–6,** 157
Smallpox, **156**
Smear test, **156**
Smell, 85
Smoking, 68, 105, 107, 111, 112,
113, 115, 117, 118, 119, 130, 132,
136, 138, 145, 147, **156,** 159, 161,
162
Snakebite, **41–2**
Snoring, 102, **156**
Soft sore *see* Chancroid
Sore throat, 7, 107, 116, 118, 123,
125, 132, 136, 138, 140, 151, 152,
156, 158, 160
what to do, **95**
Spastic colon *see* Irritable bowel
syndrome
Spina bifida, **156–7**
Spine
fractured, 29, 30–1, 107
see also Backache, Back injuries,
Bent or curved back, Hunchback,
Slipped disc *and* Spondylitis and
spondylosis
Spitting of blood, **108**
Splinter, **42**
Splints, 21, 30, 31, 35
Spondylitis and spondylosis, 105,
108, 147, **157**
Sports and fitness, 45, 46, **59–61,**
70–1
Sprain, **42, 157**
Stab wounds, 42
Sterility, caused by mumps, 142
Sterilization, contraceptive, 117,
118
Stiff neck, 97, 127, 132, 140, 147,
157
Stillbirth, 156, **157**
Stings, 11, 20, **42–3**
jellyfish, 43
plant, 42
see also Insect bites and stings
Stitch, **43**
Stomach ache, 93, 128, 132, **157**
what to do, **92**
see also Abdominal pain,
Appendicitis *and* Indigestion

Stone
   in gall-bladder, 129
   in kidney, 116, 137, **157**, 163
Storage of medicines, 6, 66
Strep throat, 156, **158**, 160
Stress, 68
Stretchers *see* Splints
Stroke, 46, 74, 105, 108, 109, 115,
   125, 136, 145, **158**, 159, 163
Sty, 43, 126, **158**
Sunbathing, 48
Sunburn, 7, **43**, 48, 59
Sunstroke *see* Heat stroke
Survival techniques, 45, 58, **61–5**
   in cold, 37, 62–3
   and escape, 64–5
   in heat and drought, 63
   in a hold-up or hijack, 64
   kits, 58, **59**, 61–2, 65
   signals, 65
   in thunderstorms, 64
   in water, 63–4
   in the wild, 64–5
Swimming, 43, 48, **60**, 61, 63, 71,
   144, 145
Symptoms: Charts of what to do,
   91–100
   backache, 98
   chest pain, 95
   constipation, 92
   cough, 96
   deafness, 96
   diarrhea, 93
   dizziness, 91
   earache, 94
   fever, 94
   headache, 97
   heavy periods, 99
   increased urination, 99
   painful joints, 97
   painful periods, 98
   rash, 100
   sore or red eye, 100
   sore throat, 95
   stomach ache, 92
   vomiting, 93
Syncope *see* Fainting
Synovitis, 112, **158**, 166
Syphilis, 114, 157, **158**, 164

T

Taste, 85
Teeth
   broken, 26
   care of the, 73, 75, 107, 130
   decayed, 107, 130, 131
   infected, 155
   see also Toothache
Teething, **159**
Temperature *see* Fever
Temperature, how to take the, 72
   see also Thermometers
Tendinitis *see* Tenosynovitis
Tennis elbow, 112
Tenosynovitis, 158, **159**
Tetanus, 118, **159**
   immunization, 19, 21, 22, 29, 42,
   47, 134, 135, 159, 172
Thermometers, 7, 48, 72
Throat, sore *see* Sore throat
Thrombosis, 68, 105, 108, 115, 117,

132, 147, 158, **159**, 164, 168–9
   coronary *see* Heart attack
Thrush *see* Moniliasis
Thumb sucking, **159**
Thyroid problems, 75, 144, 145,
   160, 171
Ticks, 38, 162
Tinea, **106**, **160**, 169
Toenail, ingrowing, **160**
Tonsillitis, 145, 156, 158, **160–1**
Toothache, 26, 125, 130, **161**
Tourniquets, 19, 42
Tracheitis, **161**
Trailers, **55–7**
Travel
   fitness to, 27, **46–8**, 145
   immunization, **47**, **134–5**, 172,
   184–5
   insurance, 48, 50, 184–5
   sickness, 7, 43, 46, 48, 143, **161**,
   165–6, 169–70
   time zones, 46
   see also Air travel, Car travel,
   Country-by-country medical and
   motoring requirements, Sea travel
   and Survival techniques
Traveller's diarrhea, 48, 59, 122,
   161, 169
Trichomoniasis *see* Vaginitis
Tropical illnesses, 47
Tuberculosis, 103, 108, 134, 150,
   161–2
   immunization, 135, 162, 172
Tumour, 103, 110, 112–13, 133,
   162, 164–5
Typhoid, 121, 128, **162**
   immunization, 47, 135, 172,
   184–5
Typhus, 138, **162**
   immunization, 47, 135, 162, 172

U

Ulcer, 101, 136, 139, **162**, 164
   bedsore, 107
   chancre, **114**
   chancroid, **114**
   eye, 108
   mouth, 26, **163**
   peptic, 147, 156, 162, 170
   Raynaud's phenomenon, **151**
   rodent, **151**
   stomach, 68, 103, 104
   varicose vein, **164**
Ulcerative colitis, 112, 116, 127
Unconsciousness, 11, 18, 25, 27, 36,
   37, 40, 41, 43–4, 104, 126
   diabetic coma, 27, 122, 169
Urethra and urethritis, 89, 131, 135,
   144, 146, 149
Urinary system, 81, 89
   see also Bladder, Kidneys,
   Prostate problems *and* Urethra
   and urethritis
Urination
   frequent, 98, 101, 107, 119, 122,
   127, 138, 149, 150, 157, **163**
   frequent/increased, what to do, **99**
   painful, 115, 131, 144, 149, 150,
   163
   see also Bedwetting *and*
   Incontinence

Urine
  blood in, 99, 112, 119, 137, 143,
    149, 157, **163**
  discoloration of, 129, **163**
  pus in, 137
  retention of, 44, 149, **163**
Urticaria *see* Nettle rash
Uterus, 90, 114, 120, 126, 127, 135,
  146, 164
  prolapse of the, 75, 135, **149**, 163

V

Vacations, and health and safety, 9,
  45–65, 66, 161, 184–5
Vagina
  bleeding from the, 38, 112, 128,
    141–2, **163–4**
  discharge from the, 98, 118, 131,
    142, 144, 152, **164**
  flooding, **127–8**
  moniliasis, **142**, 143, 164, 167,
    169
  spermicidal creams, 117, 118
Vaginismus, 153
Vaginitis, 119, 120, 152, 153, **164**,
  166
Varicella *see* Chickenpox
Varicose veins, 21, 32, 115, 117, 147,
  159, **164**
  burst, 21, 164
Variola *see* Smallpox
Vasectomy, 117
Veins, 86
  phlebitis, 115, **147**, 159
  varicose, 21, 32, 115, 117, 147,
    159, 164
  see also Thrombosis
Venereal diseases, 133, 138, 146,
  148, 152, 153, **164**
  see also A.I.D.S., Chancroid,
    Gonorrhea, Granuloma inguinale,
    Herpes genitalis,
    Lymphogranuloma venereum,
    Moniliasis, Nonspecific
    urethritis, Scabies, Syphilis *and*
    Vaginitis
Verrucas, **164–5**
Vertebrae *see* Spine
Vertigo, 91

Vitamins, 68, 69, 104, 107, 109, 115,
  121, 136, 144, 148, 151, **165**, 167
Vomiting, 26, 27, 29, 37, 44, 72, 92,
  93, 97, 101, 104, 105, 115, 116,
  122, 124, 125, 127, 128, 129, 130,
  132, 137, 140, 141, 143, 147, 150,
  157, 162, **165–6**, 167, 172
  in babies, 26, 29, **166**
  inducing, 40
  what to do, **93**
Voyeurism, 154
Vulva
  itching, 137, 164
  red and swollen, 144
Vulvitis, **166**

W

Warts, 112, **164–5**
Water contamination, 48, 59, 115,
  124, 161, 162, 167
Water on the knee, **166**
Waterskiing, 60
Water sports, **60–1**
Wax, 120, 145, **166–7**
Weight chart, 70
Wen, **119**
Whitlow, **167**
Whooping cough, 119, 166, **167**
  immunization, 134, 135, 172
Wind, 116, 128, **167**
Winding, 44
Winter sports, **59–60**
Womb *see* Uterus
Worms, 104, 137, **167**
Wounds, cleaning and dressing, 7,
  8, 19, 21, 22, 23
  see also Bleeding
Writer's cramp, 119

Y

Yellow fever, 137, **167**
  immunization, 47, 135, 167, 172
Yoga, 71

Z

Zip-fastener injuries, 44

Country-by-country medical and

	Algeria	Austria	Belgium	Cyprus	Denmark	Finland	France	Germany (W)	Great Britain	Greece
MEDICAL										
Immunizations[1]										
Cholera R										
Hepatitis R										
Malaria[1] R										
Poliomyelitis R										
Typhoid R			R							R
Reciprocal health care[2]	A	A		A	A	A	A	A		
MOTORING										
Alcohol[3] mg/100ml blood 80	80	80		80	50	80	80	80		50
Crash helmet C	C	R		C		C	C	C	C	
Seat belts C	C	C		C	C	C	C	C	C	
Disabled permits[4] A	A		A			A	A	A		
First aid kit C									C	
Warning triangles C	C	C	2C	C		C	C		C	
Driver's license–USA C	C	C	C	C	C	C	C	C	C	
–International										
Speed limits[5]										
Town mph 37	31	37	30	37	31	37	31	30	31	
kph 60	50	60	48	60	50	60	50	48	50	
Country mph	62	56	50	50	50	56	62	60	50	
kph	100	90	80	80	80	90	100	96	80	
Four-lane highway mph	62	56	60	50	50	68	80	70	50	
kph	100	90	96	80	80	110	130	112	80	
Superhighway mph	80	74		62	74	80	80	70	62	
kph	130	120		100	120	130	130	112	100	

C =Compulsory   2C= Two compulsory

1. **Immunizations** (see p.134). Discuss these with your doctor. Requirements vary from country to country. Malaria may occur in certain areas of the relevant countries indicated above.

2. **Reciprocal health care** is of varying standard. Most major medical health-care plans and most major hospital insurance programs will reimburse the insured for medical expenses incurred while travelling. These expenses must be fully documented and authenticated in the country where treatment is given. You are strongly advised to have full medical insurance when travelling abroad.

3. **Alcohol and driving.** Regulations vary but you are advised not to drink and drive. Illegal levels are given in milligrams of alcohol in 100ml blood.

4. **Disabled persons** with special parking permits may be able to use them abroad. Inquire locally when you arrive.

5. **Speed limits** may vary. Watch for speed signs and observe them. Many countries have on-the-spot fines.

motoring requirements

Ireland	Israel	Italy	Luxembourg	Malta	Morocco	Netherlands	Norway	Portugal	Spain	Sweden	Switzerland	Tunisia	Turkey	Yugoslavia
	R		R								R	R		
			R								R			
			R								R	R		
	R	R	R			R					R	R		R
	R	R	R	R			R	R			R	R		R
A		A	A		A	A	A			A				A
80			80			50	50	50	80	50	80			50
C		R	C	R	C	C	C	C	C	C	C	C	C	C
C	C	R	C		C	C	C	C	C	C	C			C
		A	A			A			A					
											R			C
	C	C	C	C	R	C	C	C	C	R	C		2C	C
C	C	C	C		C	C	C	C	C	C	C	C		C
	C	R							R		R	C		
30	31	31	37	25		31	31	37	37	31	37	31	31	37
48	50	50	60	40		50	50	60	60	50	60	50	50	60
55	50	D	56	40		50	50	56	56	43	62	62	56	50
88	80	D	90	64		80	80	90	90	70	100	100	90	80
55	60	D	56			50	50	56	62	43	62	62	56	62
88	96	D	90			80	80	90	100	70	100	100	90	100
55		D	74			62	56	74	74	62	80	74	56	74
88		D	120			100	90	120	120	110	130	120	90	120

R = Recommended   **A** = Available   **D** = Dependant on engine size

International emergency signs

Familiarize yourself with the following three signs, all of which are in international use.

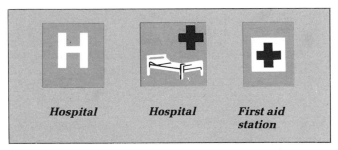

Hospital   *Hospital*   *First aid station*

In West Germany do not be confused by the following sign:

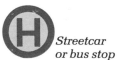

Streetcar or bus stop

Family medical records

Name of family member	
Date of birth	
Blood type	
Health service number/category/ registration/etc.	
Medical insurance details	
Serious illnesses, disorders and injuries, with dates	
Last hospital treatment for*	
date*	
Chronic or permanent illness	
X-rays, date of last for* chest	
other	
Immunization, date for last for* tetanus	
diphtheria	
whooping cough	
poliomyelitis	
measles	
German measles (rubella)	
BCG (tuberculosis)	
typhoid	
other	1
2	3
Medicine taken regularly*	1
2	3
4	5
Known allergies	
Next gynecological check due*	
Next dental check due*	
Psychiatric information	
Other information	

* Write in pencil

Name of family member	
Date of birth	
Blood type	
Health service number/category/ registration/etc.	
Medical insurance details	
Serious illnesses, disorders and injuries, with dates	
Last hospital treatment for*	
date*	
Chronic or permanent illness	
X-rays, date of last for* chest	
other	
Immunization, date for last for* tetanus	
diphtheria	
whooping cough	
poliomyelitis	
measles	
German measles (rubella)	
BCG (tuberculosis)	
typhoid	
other	1
2	3
Medicine taken regularly*	1
2	3
4	5
Known allergies	
Next gynecological check due*	
Next dental check due*	
Psychiatric information	
Other information	

* Write in pencil

Family medical records

Name of family member	
Date of birth	
Blood type	
Health service number/category/ registration/etc.	
Medical insurance details	
Serious illnesses, disorders and injuries, with dates	
Last hospital treatment for*	
date*	
Chronic or permanent illness	
X-rays, date of last for* chest	
other	
Immunization, date for last for* tetanus	
diphtheria	
whooping cough	
poliomyelitis	
measles	
German measles (rubella)	
BCG (tuberculosis)	
typhoid	
other	1
2	3
Medicine taken regularly*	1
2	3
4	5
Known allergies	
Next gynecological check due*	
Next dental check due*	
Psychiatric information	
Other information	

* Write in pencil

Name of family member	
Date of birth	
Blood type	
Health service number/category/ registration/etc.	
Medical insurance details	
Serious illnesses, disorders and injuries, with dates	
Last hospital treatment for*	
date*	
Chronic or permanent illness	
X-rays, date of last for* chest	
other	
Immunization, date for last for* tetanus	
diphtheria	
whooping cough	
poliomyelitis	
measles	
German measles (rubella)	
BCG (tuberculosis)	
typhoid	
other	1
2	3
Medicine taken regularly*	1
2	3
4	5
Known allergies	
Next gynecological check due*	
Next dental check due*	
Psychiatric information	
Other information	

* Write in pencil

Family medical records

Name of family member	
Date of birth	
Blood type	
Health service number/category/registration/etc.	
Medical insurance details	
Serious illnesses, disorders and injuries, with dates	
Last hospital treatment for*	
date*	
Chronic or permanent illness	
X-rays, date of last for* chest	
other	
Immunization, date for last for* tetanus	
diphtheria	
whooping cough	
poliomyelitis	
measles	
German measles (rubella)	
BCG (tuberculosis)	
typhoid	
other	1
2	3
Medicine taken regularly*	1
2	3
4	5
Known allergies	
Next gynecological check due*	
Next dental check due*	
Psychiatric information	
Other information	

* Write in pencil

Emergency chart

Home address and tel. no.
Exact location of home (to be completed as it is easier to read it out in an emergency than to try to describe it)
Name, address and tel. no. of nearest relatives: 1
2
Name, address and tel. no. of neighbor/friend
Doctor (day)
Doctor (night): tel. no.
Alternative doctor
Pharmacist
Dentist
Local emergency hospital
Other hospital

Dial 911 for POLICE, FIRE, AMBULANCE

Emergency chart

Specialists: 1
2
Name and tel. no. of priest/minister/rabbi
Welfare services: 1
2
3
Vet
Name, address and tel. no. of employer: Office
Home: tel. no.
Employees: 1
2
Weather forecast: tel. no.
Taxi – 24-hour service: tel. nos.
Utility company – tel. nos: Water
Electricity
Gas
Telephone
Medical and hospital insurance company
Policy no.